PAU-OL6-CTP3
Preparation Agenda for Study Success

ULTRA P.A.S.S.
Adult Echocardiography
Registry Review Workbook
4ᵗʰ Edition

Featuring the On-Line Media Center
Containing Video Clips and Audio Narration

Written by

Christie Jordan, BS, RDCS, RCS, RCIS, FASE

Edited by
Lori Green, BA, RT, RDMS, RDCS, RVT

Published by:

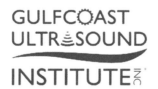
GULFCOAST
ULTRASOUND
INSTITUTE INC.

111 2nd Ave. NE Suite 800
St. Petersburg, FL 33701
Tel: (727)363-4500
Fax: (727)363-0811
www.gcus.com

The Gulfcoast Ultrasound Institute, Inc.® is accredited by the Accreditation Council for Continuing Medical Education to provide continuing medical education for physicians.

The Gulfcoast Ultrasound Institute, Inc.® designates this enduring material for a maximum of **20.0 AMA PRA Category 1 Credits™**. Physicians should claim only the credit commensurate with the extent of their participation in the activity.

LENGTH OF MATERIALS:
The estimated time to review all sections is approximately 16.5 hours. A post-lecture quiz should be completed after reviewing each section; Estimated time to complete all section quiz questions: 3.0 hours. Estimated time to complete online CME quiz: 1/2 hour. Total estimated time to complete the workbook activity as designed: 20 hours.

EDUCATIONAL NEEDS STATEMENT:
The planning committee has determined a need for this educational activity based on request from the medical community, expanded utilization of ultrasound, certification and lab accreditation requirements.

ENDURING MATERIALS COURSE OBJECTIVES:
Please see opening statements at each section.

RELEASE INFORMATION: See Back Cover

Author: Christie Jordan, BS, RDCS, RCS, RCIS, FASE
Cardiovascular Technology Faculty Program Director
Florida State College at Jacksonville, Jacksonville, Florida
No relevant financial relationships to disclose

Disclosure of Individuals in Control of Content
In addition to the faculty listed the following individuals are recognized by GUI as being in control of content of this program:

James Mateer, MD, RDMS (Medical Director-planner & QI Task Force)
Medical Director, Gulfcoast Ultrasound Institute
Milwaukee, WI
No relevant financial relationships to disclose

Charlotte Derr, MD, RDMS, FACEP (Co-Medical Director-planner & QI Task Force)
Assistant Professor of Emergency Medicine &
Fellowship Director of Emergency Medicine
Ultrasound Fellowship Program
University of South Florida Medical School
Tampa, FL
No relevant financial relationships to disclose

Andreas Dewitz, MD, RDMS (Member of Advisory Board & QI Task Force Subcommittee)
Associate Professor of Emergency MedicineVice Chair of Ultrasound Education
Boston Medical Center
Boston, MA
No relevant financial relationships to disclose

Lori Green, BA, RT, RDMS, RDCS, RVT (Program Director-planner, Content Reviewer, QI Task Force)
Gulfcoast Ultrasound Institute, Inc.
St. Petersburg, FL
No relevant financial relationships to disclose

Trisha Reo, AAS, RDMS, RVT (Program Coordinator-planner, Content Reviewer, QI Task Force)
Gulfcoast Ultrasound Institute, Inc.
St. Petersburg, FL
No relevant financial relationships to disclose

PAU-OL6-CTP3
ULTRA P.A.S.S. Adult Echocardiography Registry Review Workbook
ISBN# 978-1-950973-37-8   **11/18/2019**

ADULT ECHOCARDIOGRAPHY REGISTRY REVIEW WORKBOOK
TABLE OF CONTENTS

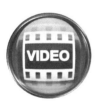

When you see this Video Screen Icon in a chapter paragraph,
play the indicated video clip from the **On-line Media Center**.
You can view them on your computer/smartphone or web-enabled device

1. Point your browser to https://www.gcus.com
2. Log into your account
3. Select "My Activities" from the top menu
4. Click the "Media Center" button for PAU-OL6-CTP3

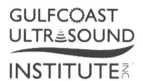

Section 1:

Anatomy and Physiology

Section 1: ANATOMY AND PHYSIOLOGY

Objectives

Upon completion of this module you should be able to:

- Recognize and describe cardiac anatomy and physiology
- Identify the subdivisions of the ventricles
- State the normal pressures in all four cardiac chambers
- Compare electrical and mechanical systole
- Relate the filling phases of diastole to the cardiac cycle
- Compare timing of cardiac events to ECG
- Identify basic heart sounds

ANATOMY AND PHYSIOLOGY

SEGMENTS OF THE HEART

Right Atrium

The heart receives deoxygenated blood from the venous system that returns this deoxygenated blood to the right side of the heart. This blood empties into the right atrium via the superior vena cava, inferior vena cava, and the coronary sinus.

The **superior and inferior vena cava** returns blood from the upper and lower regions of the body respectively. The **coronary sinus** drains deoxygenated blood from the heart. The superior and inferior vena cava enter the right atrium infero-posteriorly and supero-posteriorly. The inferior vena cava has a rudimentary valve formed by a tissue fold called the Eustachian valve. The superior vena cava has no such valve. The coronary sinus enters the right atrium between the IVC and the tricuspid valve. It is guarded by a flap of tissue which forms a rudimentary valve called the Thebesian valve.

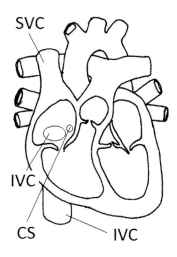

Right-sided anatomy of the heart

The **right atrium** is located on the right, superior portion of the heart and forms the right lateral cardiac border. It is located behind and to the right of the right ventricle and lies mostly anterior to the left atrium. The right atrium can be divided into two sections: 1) a smooth section, and 2) a rough, trabeculated section. The smooth area of the right atrium is located posteriorly where the great vessels (SVC and IVC) enter the right atrium. The trabeculated area of the right atrium that is usually composed of pectinate muscles houses the right atrial appendage which extends from the right atrium and drapes over the aortic root. The appendage is a triangular shaped pouch like structure with a large orifice. Its purpose is to increase the size of the right atrium so it can hold a greater volume of blood.

From the right atrium blood passes through the **tricuspid valve.** The tricuspid valve is made up of three leaflets: 1) anterior, 2) septal (medial) and 3) posterior. This area is also called the **right ventricular inflow tract** as it directs blood into the right ventricle.

Right Ventricle

Once blood crosses the tricuspid valve it enters the **right ventricle**. The RV is typically the most anterior cardiac chamber and appears somewhat crescent shaped. The walls of the right ventricle are much thinner as compared to the walls of the left ventricle. The right ventricle walls are also lined with trabeculae carnae.

Both ventricles share the interventricular septum as their medial wall. The moderator band is a muscle commonly seen during an echocardiogram and is located in the right ventricle. The moderator band extends from the lower interventricular septum to the anterior wall, and then joins the anterior papillary muscle.

The **right ventricular outflow tract** is also called the conus arteriosus or infundibulum. The crista supraventricularis, a thick muscle, separates the outflow tract from the inflow tract. The supraventricularis arches over the anterior leaflet of the tricuspid valve. The right ventricular outflow tract extends from the tricuspid annulus to the pulmonic valve. From the right ventricular outflow tract, blood crosses the **pulmonic valve** and enters into the pulmonary artery. The pulmonic valve is made up of three cusps: 1) anterior, 2) right and 3) left cusps.

The **pulmonary artery** returns deoxygenated blood to the lungs. The pulmonary artery begins at the pulmonic valve level where it bifurcates into the right and left pulmonary arteries a few centimeters from its origin. The pulmonary artery has thinner walls in adults, with pressures approximately one-sixth of the systemic circulation in the normal adult heart. Pulmonary capillary pressures at rest are only 7-10 mmHg as opposed to systemic capillary pressures which are 25 to 35 mmHg.

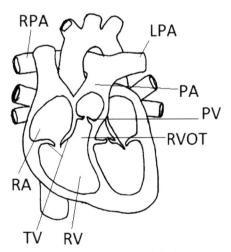

Right-sided anatomy of the heart

Left Atrium

The **atria** are the receiving chambers for blood in the heart. The left atrium receives

oxygenated blood from the pulmonary veins. There are normally four or five **pulmonary veins.** The left atrium also acts as a reservoir of the heart for ventricular systole, provides a significant amount of blood to the left ventricle during left atrial contraction, and is a conduit during left ventricular filling.

The **left atrium** lies superior and posterior to the other cardiac structures, and is slightly smaller than the right atrium although they have about the same thickness. The left atrial appendage is a projection of the left atrium from the anterolateral surface alongside the pulmonary artery. The left atrial appendage contains pectinate muscles while the rest of the left atrium does not. It is finger shaped and its opening has a narrow orifice. Like the right atrial appendage, its purpose is to increase the size of the left atrium to allow for an increase of volume blood flow. The left atrial appendage is an area that is of concern in patients with slow blood flow or in atrial fibrillation as this is a common area for blood clots to form.

The **left ventricular inflow tract** is funnel shaped and formed by the mitral annulus, mitral leaflets, and chordae tendineae. The inflow tract directs blood from the left atrium to the left ventricle inferiorly and anteriorly.

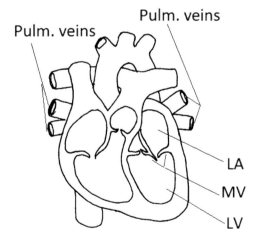

Left-sided anatomy of the heart

Left Ventricle

Once blood crosses the mitral valve it enters the **left ventricle.** The left ventricle is the larger of the two ventricles yet both the right and the left eject equal amounts of blood volume. It is the thickest chamber the heart containing about 75% of the muscle mass of the entire heart and forms the apex of the heart. The left ventricle has an ellipsoid or conical shape and contains trabeculae carneae, although the left ventricular septal surface is smoother than the right ventricular septal surface which is heavily trabeculated.

The **left ventricular outflow tract** is surrounded by the inferior surface of the anteromedial mitral leaflet, the interventricular septum, and the left ventricular free wall. It ends at the level of the aortic annulus.

Blood passes from the left ventricle through the **aortic valve**. The aortic valve contains three cusps: 1) right coronary 2) left coronary and 3) non-coronary cusps. The names of the cusp are derived by where the coronaries arise off of the aorta in the sinus of valsalva area.

After the blood crosses the aortic valve it enters the aortic root where the oxygenated blood is distributed to the body. The initial area of the aorta is called the ascending aorta then arches around to form the arch of the aorta and into the descending aorta which runs down the body before bifurcating. There are three main branches at the arch area of the aorta 1) innominate or brachiocephalic which branches into the right subclavian and right common carotid arteries, 2) left common carotid and the 3) left subclavian branch.

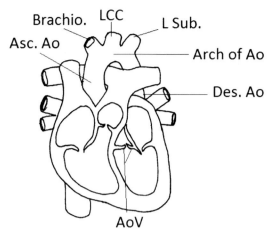

Left sided anatomy of the heart

The set of heart valves that separate the atria from the ventricles are called the **atrioventricular valves**. These are the mitral and tricuspid valves. The tricuspid valve regulates flow between the right atrium and right ventricle. There are three leaflets composed of fibrous tissue covered by endocardium. The tricuspid orifice is larger than the mitral. The tricuspid leaflets are not equal in size. The anterior leaflet is the largest and extends from the infundibular region to the inferolateral right ventricular wall. The medial leaflet is the septal leaflet. It attaches to both the membranous and muscular interventricular septa. The posterior leaflet is usually the smallest and attaches to the tricuspid ring.

The **mitral leaflets** are similar in structure to the **tricuspid leaflets**, but are thicker due to the higher pressures of the left ventricle This is necessary to withstand the higher pressures in the left ventricle. The leaflets are attached at one end to the annulus fibrosis which completely circles the valve orifice. There are two mitral leaflets, the anteromedial leaflet is triangular in shape and extends from the posteromedial left ventricle to the anterolateral left ventricular wall. This leaflet is continuous with the posterior aortic root wall.

The posterolateral mitral leaflet is longer and circles approximately two thirds of the mitral valve orifice. It attaches to the annulus fibrosus superiorly. (The leaflets are usually referred to as the anterior and posterior leaflets in the clinical setting.) There are usually two groups of papillary muscles in the left ventricle located below the anterolateral and posteromedial commissure.

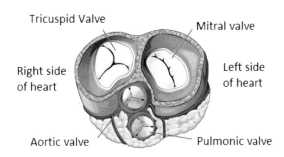

Heart Valves

Chordae tendineae and papillary muscles are located in both the right and left ventricles

There are usually three papillary muscles in the right ventricle, which have strong chords of fibrous tissue called **chordae tendineae** arising from their tips. The chordae attach the valve leaflets to the papillary muscles. The **papillary muscles** pull the valve leaflets together and downward during isovolumetric ventricular contractions. The tricuspid valve is usually more apically located than the mitral valve and has chordal attachments to the interventricular septum

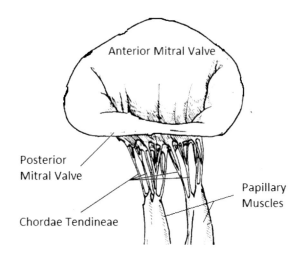

Chordae Tendineae and Papillary Muscles

The other set of valves are referred to as the **semilunar valves** and consists of the pulmonic and aortic valves. Both valves are made up of three crescent moon-shaped cusps hence the name "semilunar". The aortic valve is in the left ventricular outflow tract and the pulmonic valve is in the right ventricular outflow tract. The valves are similar in appearance in that they are made up of three fibrous cusps. The ends of each cusp have an arantius nodule which helps to support the cusp and prevent leakage of blood from the valve to the ventricle. The area around the nodules of arantius can become thickened and calcific as a patient ages.

Subdivisions of Ventricles

The coronary or atrioventricular sulcus is the external separation of the atria from the ventricles. The coronary sulcus circles the heart between the ventricles and atria.

The ventricles are defined externally by the interventricular sulci which extends down from the coronary sulcus to the apex. The atria are defined externally by a groove between the right pulmonary veins and vena cava on the posterior surface.

The crux of the heart is the location where the coronary sulcus meets the interventricular sulcus. It is at this point internally that the interatrial septum joins the interventricular septum.

The internal partition of the right and left ventricles is called the interventricular septum. The interventricular septum is primarily muscular, except for the membranous septum. The membranous septum lies slightly inferior to the right and non-coronary cusps of the aorta. The upper third of the interventricular septum is smooth endocardium. The bulk of the septum and left ventricular wall are lined by the trabeculae carneae.

LAYERS OF THE HEART WALL

The walls of the ventricles have three distinct layers, the **epicardium** or external layer, the **myocardium** or middle layer, and the **endocardium** or inner layer. The blood supply to the walls of the heart is via the coronary arteries. The coronary arteries traverse the epicardium before entering the myocardium.

The **myocardium** is the cardiac muscle responsible for the hearts ability to contract. The myocardium is composed of interlacing bundles of cardiac muscle fibers. The myocardial thickness varies with each chamber. The left ventricle is the thickest and is usually three times thicker than the right ventricle. The right ventricle has a moderately thick myocardium, while the atria have fairly thin walls. Cardiac muscle beats for a lifetime without long rest periods.

The **endocardium** of the heart forms the inner surface of the myocardium and is composed of a thin layer of endothelial tissue.

The **epicardium** is the visceral layer of the pericardium and the outer most layer of the heart wall.

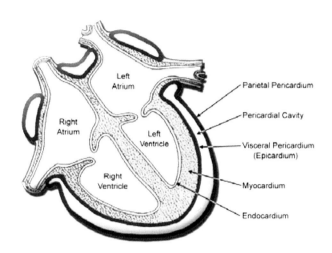

Left Atrium

Right Atrium

Left Ventricle

Right Ventricle

Parietal Pericardium

Pericardial Cavity

Visceral Pericardium (Epicardium)

Myocardium

Endocardium

Layers of Heart Wall/Pericardium

LAYERS OF THE PERICARDIUM

There is a membrane that surrounds the heart, serves as protection, and holds the heart in its place. This membrane is called the **pericardium**. The pericardium consists of two main parts: 1) **fibrous** layer which is the outer layer and 2) the **serous** layer. The fibrous layer is a tough fibrotic sac that surrounds the heart and anchors the heart in the mediastinum. The serous layer is a thinner layer that consists of two layers: 1) parietal and 2) visceral layers. The parietal layer is fused to the fibrous pericardium and the visceral layer is the inner most layer of the pericardium and also the outermost layer of the heart wall (epicardium).

Between the parietal and visceral layers of the pericardium lies the pericardial sac. This sac contains a small amount of serous fluid which serves as a lubricant for the heart.

15

The pericardium attaches at the base to the diaphragm, apex, and goes as far as the first subdivision of the great vessels. Anteriorly, the pericardium attaches to the sternum. The lateral attachment of the pericardium is to the mediastinal pleura, while attaching posteriorly to the esophagus, trachea, and principal bronchi.

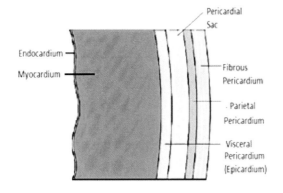

Layers of the pericardium

GREAT VESSELS

The **embryonic truncus arteriosus** is the origin of both the aorta and the pulmonary artery. In the adult the aorta's walls are much thicker than the pulmonary artery walls. At birth the wall thickness of both vessels are similar.

The arteries have three tissue layers. The inner layer is a single cell thickness of endothelial cells and is called the tunica intima. The middle layer is a thicker muscle layer called the tunica media and the outer layer is a white fibrous layer called the tunica adventitia. As the arteries branch out they become smaller and are referred to as arterioles. Arterioles have only two layer walls; the tunica media and intima. These will continue to branch and thin, eventually

becoming the capillaries. Capillaries have only intima as their walls. The capillaries have the ability to expand and contract based on the blood supply need to an area. The capillaries anastomose with the venous system.

The **aorta** carries oxygenated blood away from the heart during left ventricular systole while the pulmonary artery carries deoxygenated blood to the lungs. Typically, it is stated that arteries are oxygenated blood and veins are deoxygenated blood. With the heart, arteries carry blood away from the heart and veins bring blood back to the heart. The pulmonary artery carries blood away from the heart yet holds deoxygenated blood. Pulmonary veins bring oxygenated blood back to the heart.

The aorta is divided into distinctive areas, the sinuses of Valsalva which lie adjacent to the coronary cusps, the sinotubular junction which is the area where the sinuses connect to the ascending aorta, the ascending aorta, the transverse aortic arch and the descending aorta. The aorta continues into the thoracic aorta and the abdominal aorta. The thoracic aorta becomes the abdominal aorta after it penetrates the diaphragm. The aortic arch has three main branches: the innominate or brachiocephalic artery, the left common carotid artery, and the left subclavian artery. Variations of the branching of these vessels may occur.

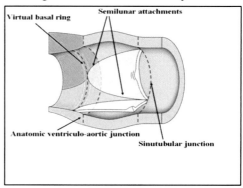

16

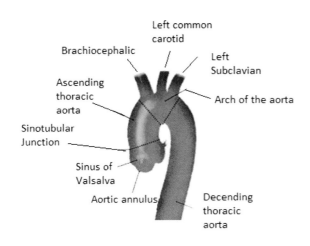

Left common carotid

Brachiocephalic

Left Subclavian

Ascending thoracic aorta

Arch of the aorta

Sinotubular Junction

Sinus of Valsalva

Aortic annulus

Decending thoracic aorta

Areas of the Aorta

The two main coronary arteries are the right and left coronary arteries which arise from the region of the coronary cusp in the sinuses of Valsalva. The myocardium is perfused from the epicardium to the endocardium.

Coronary artery flow can be influenced by coronary artery disease, heart rate, and diastolic pressures in the aortic root and left ventricle. The myocardium is perfused mainly during diastole. When the aortic valve is closed, the sinuses of Valsalva become engorged and the myocardium is non-contractile.

Coronary Sinus vs. Descending Aorta

The coronary sinus appears as an echo free structure located in the region of the posterior atrioventricular groove. Typically, if the coronary sinus is identified on the ultrasound exam, it is small and contained within the cardiac tissue on the parasternal long axis view. However, the coronary sinus may appear dilated in the setting of a persistent left superior vena cava.

The descending aorta is seen on multiple views, but should be differentiated from the coronary sinus in the parasternal long axis view. The descending aorta is larger than the normal coronary sinus. The descending aorta lies inferior to the left atrium and the region of the atrioventricular groove and lies outside the pericardial shadow. In the parasternal long axis view, the descending aorta is used to help differentiate between pericardial or pleural effusions.

Coronary Arteries

The blood supply to the heart muscle itself is via the <u>coronary arteries</u> which are branches of the aortic root.

The **<u>right coronary artery</u>** arises from the anterior (right) coronary sinus and courses between the pulmonary artery, right atrium and right ventricle. It curves around the right border of the heart and continues on the posterior aspect to the posterior interventricular groove. At this juncture, the right coronary artery divides into two branches, the transverse branch and the descending branch. These branches anastomose with the left coronary artery. The obtuse marginal branch is also a branch that arises from the right coronary artery distal to the bifurcation.

The right coronary artery usually supplies blood to the inferior wall, the basal interventricular septum, the basal posterior wall and the right ventricular free wall. There may be two ostia in the region of the right coronary artery. Besides the ostium for the right coronary artery itself, the conus artery may arise here as a separate artery. The conus artery is an important branch since it may serve as a collateral. If the conus artery does not have its own ostium, it is the first branch of the right coronary artery.

The **<u>left coronary artery</u>** divides into the left anterior descending and the left circumflex arteries. There are one to three branches that can arise from the left main coronary artery.

17

These branches lie diagonally over the free wall between the left anterior descending and the left circumflex arteries. They are referred to as the **diagonal left ventricular branches**.

The **left anterior descending artery** usually feeds the apex, basal, mid interventricular septum, and the anterior walls. The **left circumflex** feeds the mid and basal lateral walls, and the mid posterior wall. Although not well visualized ultrasonically, the coronary arteries are sometimes imaged at their origins when performing a parasternal short axis view at the aortic valve level and on the apical four or five chamber views.

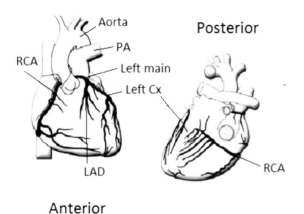

Coronary Anatomy

Coronary Veins

Deoxygenated blood from the heart tissues is returned via the coronary veins. There are three coronary vein systems. The smallest is the **thebesian veins** and are usually located in the right atrium and right ventricle.

The **anterior cardiac veins** are the second largest of the three sets of veins and drain most of the right ventricle.

The third and largest venous system is the **coronary sinus** and its branches. This system becomes the great cardiac vein near the origin of the anterior descending artery.

The **great cardiac vein** anastomoses with a smaller vein called the **oblique vein of Marshall.** An incompetent valve exists here and marks the anatomic division of the great cardiac vein and the coronary sinus. The coronary sinus courses along the posterior wall of the left atrium and extends into the right atrium of the heart where the venous blood is returned. The coronary sinus is guarded by another incompetent valve called the Thebesian valve. The coronary sinus may be seen on the ultrasound exam usually in a parasternal long axis view and possibly in the apical two chamber view. The coronary sinus lies in the atrioventricular groove between the left ventricular posterior wall and the left atrium. If the coronary sinus is dilated, it may be confused with the descending aorta. The descending aorta lies posterior to the heart under the left atrium and lies outside the pericardium.

Normal Pressures in Cardiac Chambers and Great Vessels

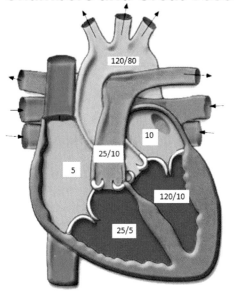

Left ventricle in systole 90 to 140 mmHg	Left ventricle end diastole 4-12 mmHg
Left atrium maximum 6-20 mmHg	Left atrium minimum -2 to +6 mmHg
Pulmonary artery systole 15-28 mmHg	Pulmonary artery diastole 5-16 mmHg
Right ventricle systole 15-28 mmHg	Right ventricle systole 0-8 mmHg
Right atrium maximum 2-14 mmHg	Right atrium minimum -2 to +6 mmHg
Vena cava maximum 2-14 mmHg	Vena cava minimum 0-8 mmHg
Aorta systole 90-140 mmHg	Aorta diastole 60-90 mmHg

CARDIAC CONDUCTION SYSTEM

The function of the electrical system of the heart is maintained primarily by two rather large nodes. These are nerve-like conduits that transmit impulses to the inner surface of the ventricles. The heart muscle is myogenic which allows for electrical stimulation. The muscle of the heart has a negative potential, but during depolarization this is lost and the muscle becomes slightly positive. This lasts only a fraction of a second before repolarization occurs and the positive ions resume their original positions.

The **sino-atrial node** is known as the primary pacemaker of the heart. The sino-atrial node has the ability to create spontaneous action potential (automaticity). The SA node is located in the posterior wall of the right atrium beneath and medial to the entry point of the superior vena cava. The SA node spreads waves of electrical excitation through the atria via the intermodal pathways and the Bachmann's Bundle. These specialized fibers relay the pulse to the **atrioventricular node** or AV node. This is the secondary pacemaker of the heart. The AV node is located posteriorly in the lower right atrium.

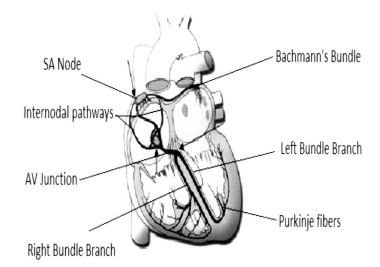

The action potential slows at the AV node to allow for mechanical ventricular filling. From the AV node the electricity spreads to the **bundle of His**. This allows conduction to reach the ventricles. After moving through the Bundle of His electricity propagates to the **right and left bundle branches**. These branches extend through the interventricular septum and run to the ventricular apex of the heart. The final spread of electricity is to the **Purkinje fibers** which spread electricity to the remaining myocardium.

When leads are placed on the body in specified places, the electrical information from the various cardiac phases can be monitored. The deflections or impulses are different for each part of the cardiac cycle. The parts on the EKG are represented by the following: the P wave, the QRS complex and the T wave.

The P wave represents atrial depolarization. Atrial contraction occurs just after the P wave. The QRS complex represents ventricular depolarization. Mechanical systole occurs shortly after the QRS complex. The T wave represents ventricular repolarization which occurs approximately 0.25 seconds after depolarization. This initiates ventricular relaxation.

Cardiac tissue is one of several tissues in the body that respond to electrical excitation. The normal heart possesses a specialized system that spontaneously generates and distributes an electrical impulse.

Propagation of Electrical Activity

The ability to spontaneously depolarize a cell membrane is called **automaticity** and exists in certain specialized cells within the heart muscle. In the normal heart, the **sinus node** is the primary pacemaker and the **His-Purkinje** system is a backup. Sinus node activation is usually between 60 and 100 beats per minute and it spreads its impulse through the atria toward the **AV node.** Once to the AV node, the pulse travels to the His bundle, then down the right and left bundles to the **Purkinje fibers** where ventricular activation is initiated. The result of this propagating impulse through the heart's conduction system is termed **excitation-contraction coupling.**

Excitation-Contraction Coupling

Excitation-contraction coupling is the link between the hearts' propagated action potential and the mechanical events of muscular contraction. The exact mechanism by which this action potential signals the muscle fibers of the myocardium to contract is unknown, but it is thought to involve the $Ca2+$ion.

How this electrical-mechanical relationship works is as follows with distinct phases:

Phase 0-1: The action potential within the hearts conduction system causes an initial rapid influx of Na+ ions. Inflow of these cells produces rapid depolarization.

Phase 2: This phase is the plateau period due to Ca+2 inflow. Ca2+ ions bind to specific sites on the contractile proteins within myocardial muscle cells. The uptake of Ca2+ ions permits muscle fibrils to contract. Also K+ channels will open and some K+ will flow out.

Phase 3: Repolarization begins when Ca2+ channels close and there is an outflow of K+.

Phase 4: Outflow of the K+ causes the cell to become negatively charged inside allowing the cell to begin the process again of depolarization. This is the resting phase.

The mechanical action of the myocardium is a dynamic event and dependent on many variables and situations

Correlation of the mechanical events dependent on the ECG is important. Rapid ventricular depolarization is seen with the QRS on the ECG and the T wave on the ECG denotes ventricular repolarization.

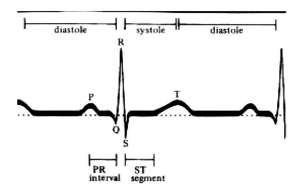

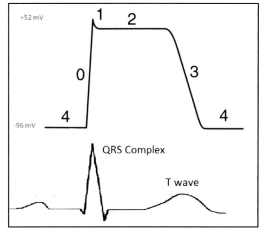

Action Potential Curve with ECG

MECHANICAL CONSIDERATIONS AND EVENTS

An attempt has been made to explain various mechanical relationships that exist and their effect on cardiac function. The first and probably most common mechanical consideration of ventricular function is termed the Frank-Starling Law.

Frank Starling Law (length-tension relationship)

This law concludes that there is a direct relationship between the degree of myocardial muscle fiber stretch and the force generated by the succeeding contraction. The degree of fiber stretch is usually, but not always related to ventricular distensibility and ventricular volume. The primary stretch of the heart muscle correlates with preload (the volume of blood that fills the chambers during diastole). The corresponding succeeding contraction correlates with stroke volume. Generally, increases in preload (fiber stretch) will result in an increase in stroke volume (succeeding contraction). Another important mechanical consideration is the Force-Velocity relationship.

Valve Opening and Closure

The opening and closing of the atrioventricular valves is dependent on the pressure differences between the atria and ventricles. When the blood moves into the atria, the pressures in the atria increase. When this pressure increases above the pressure in the ventricles, the atrioventricular valves (mitral and tricuspid) open to let the blood into the ventricles. When the pressure decreases enough, the valves will again close due to the higher pressure in the ventricles. When the pressures in the ventricles exceed the pressure in the great vessels (pulmonary artery and aorta), the semilunar valves (pulmonic and aortic) open and the blood is ejected out of the ventricles. When enough blood is ejected and the pressure decreases in the ventricles, the semilunar valves close and the cycle continues.

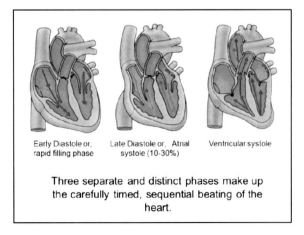

Early Diastole or,   Late Diastole or,   Atrial   Ventricular systole
rapid filling phase   systole (10-30%)

Three separate and distinct phases make up
the carefully timed, sequential beating of the
heart.

Phases of the Cardiac Cycle (Electromechanical Events)

Once the electrical activation of the heart is complete, certain mechanical considerations come into play which constitutes the muscular function of the heart. The cardiac cycle is the complete series of mechanical events that make up the function of the heart. It is divided into two periods, **diastole** (mechanical relaxation) and **systole** (mechanical contraction), and subdivided to phases.

1. Passive filling phase (ventricular diastole)
The first phase in ventricular diastole is a passive filling phase. When the pressure in the atria override the pressure in the ventricles, the AV valves open and ventricular filling begins. This phase consists of rapid and slow filling (diastasis) into the ventricles.   Seventy percent of blood that is ejected from the atrial fills the ventricular due to passive filling.

The next phase of ventricular diastole is the stage of atrial systole (beginning of propagation of electrical activity).

2. Atrial systole (p-wave on EKG; late diastole)

This phase represents active ventricular filling as a result of atrial contraction. It occurs just after the P wave on the ECG and is associated with the "a" wave on left atrial pressure tracing. Atrial systole accounts for 30% of the blood that is ejected from the atria. If a patient is in atrial fibrillation, this phase does not occur.

3. Isovolumetric contraction

Ventricular filling just occurred and the AV valves close due to the pressure in the ventricles becoming higher than that in the atrial. For a period of about .05 seconds, all fours valves are closed. Ventricular systole begins with the isovolumetric contraction and ventricular pressure increasing. When the pressure in the ventricles override the pressure in the great vessels, the semilunar valves will open.

4. Ventricular ejection

The next occurring phase is that of rapid ventricular ejection which occurs midway through the QRS on the ECG tracing. It is almost simultaneous with the opening of the aortic valve. The last phase of ventricular systole is the phase of reduced ventricular ejection. It is less well-defined than the rapid ejection phase, but would seem to correspond to the point when the left ventricular volume curve indicates a falloff in the rate of ejection, and the point just before peak systolic pressure in the left ventricle and aorta.

5. Isovolumetric relaxation

Once the pressure in the ventricles drop below the pressure in the great vessels, the semilunar valves will close. The next phase is **isovolumetric relaxation**. This phase occurs just after aortic valve and pulmonic valve closure and prior to the opening of the mitral and tricuspid valves. On the ECG tracing it occurs just after the T wave. Again, all four valves are closed and ventricular pressure is decreasing to allow the atrial pressure to override the pressure in the ventricles.

LEFT VENTRICULAR FUNCTION: INDICATORS AND NORMAL VALUES

Once the electrical-mechanical considerations of the heart are understood, an attempt must be made to quantify left ventricular performance. Certain parameters are commonly used in order to evaluate cardiac function and general conditioning of the pumping action of the heart. The descriptive terms usually used when explaining heart function are: **stroke volume, ejection fraction, cardiac output, and cardiac index.**

Stroke Volume

Stroke volume (SV) is the amount of blood pumped out of the aorta with every heartbeat. Stroke volume depends on the aortic blood pressure, the end-diastolic volume, and the contraction of the ventricle.

$$SV = TVI \times CSA$$

◆ Normal range of values is Between 32 – 58 ml/beat.

By Doppler echocardiography, stroke volume (SV) is measured as the cross-sectional area (CSA) of the valve at the level of the annulus multiplied by the time velocity integral (TVI) of the pulsed wave Doppler at the level of the valve.

Ejection Fraction

Ejection fraction (EF) is related to stroke volume and is the percentage of preload or blood filling the left ventricle that is ejected with every beat of the heart.

Ejection fraction is measured using echocardiography by 2-dimensional tracing of the endocardial borders in the modified Simpson's method.

$$EF = \frac{LVEDV - LVESV}{LVEDV} \quad X \quad 100$$

Cardiac Output

Cardiac output (CO) is the total volume of blood circulated in the body per minute. Cardiac output is measured as the stroke volume (SV) multiplied by heart rate (HR).

By Doppler echocardiography cardiac output is measured in the same way.

CO= SV x HR

◆ Normal values of this parameter fall between 4 – 6 liters/minute.

Cardiac Index

Cardiac index is defined as cardiac output adjusted by body surface area. It takes into account the size of the patient when dealing with cardiac output.

◆ Normal range is between 2.8 – 4.2 liters/minute/m^2.

PULMONARY VS. SYSTEMIC CIRCULATION: DIFFERENCES AND SIMILARITIES

In understanding cardiac physiology, it is basic to understand that the heart is really made up of two distinct, although connected circuits: the right heart or pulmonary circuit and the left heart or systemic circuit. Basic differences in the two circulations are pressure differences, level of oxygen saturation, and which area of the body each side pumps blood to.

Pressure

Intracardiac pressure is much lower on the right side of the heart being about 20% of what it is on the left.

◆ Normal range of right ventricular and pulmonary artery systolic pressure is between 15 – 25mmHg

Normal Values

Normal pressure values according to the Hurst text of the Heart are as follows:

◆ right atrium varies between 2 –14 mmHg during atrial systole and 2 – 6 mm/Hg in atrial diastole. Pressure is stated as a mean.
◆ right ventricular pressure varies between 15 – 18 mm/Hg in systole and 0 –8 mmHg in diastole
◆ left ventricular pressure varies between 100 – 140 mmHg and 3 – 12 for diastole.
◆ left atrial pressure varies between 5 -12 in systole and 1 – 10 mmHg in atrial diastole. Pressure is stated as a mean.

MANEUVERS ALTERING CARDIAC PHYSIOLOGY

There are a few basic maneuvers that alter cardiac physiology and should be used during various echocardiographic examinations.

The result of all maneuvers is to accentuate heart murmurs and heart sounds.

Valsalva maneuver is the holding of the patient's breath and bearing down, with or without the inhalation of amyl nitrate. The results of this maneuver causes positive intrathoracic pressure which diminishes venous return so that cardiac output and arterial pressure fall.
The reflex increase in sympathetic outflow causes the heart rate to increase and contracts arterioles.

Amyl nitrate -slow inhalation of amyl nitrate also causes changes in cardiac physiology and results in: vasodilatation and decreased filling of the left ventricle

These two methods are most often used to provoke a ventricular gradient in patients with hypertrophic obstructive cardiomyopathies.

Position -changing the patient position from supine to sitting or standing results in:
◆ changes the afterload and preload of blood in the system
◆ sometimes used in the assessment of mitral valve prolapse

NORMAL HEART SOUND GENERATION AND TIMING

In the normal heart, sounds are generated by the mechanical action of the valves and the muscle itself. Most individuals manifest two basic heart sounds with a third and fourth sound sometimes heard in normal individuals. The four heart sounds are designated as S1 through S4 and fall into two categories.

The first category of sounds is high frequency transients that are associated with valves opening or closing. The second type of sounds generated is low frequency sounds related to early and late diastolic filling of the ventricles.

S1 heart sound is generated by the **closure of the atrioventricular valves** shortly after the rise in pressure in the ventricles. It is broken down into two components designated M1 and T1, corresponding to the mitral and tricuspid contribution. Both components occur almost simultaneously with the mitral sound being the louder of the two and generally drowning out the tricuspid. This occurs on the R wave of the ECG.

S2 is a high frequency heart sound that is generated by the **closure of the semilunar valves** toward the end of systole. It occurs just after the T wave on the ECG tracing and is broken down into two component parts similar to the S1 sound. The two component parts of S2 are termed A2 and P2 and represent the aortic and pulmonic valve contributions to the sound generated. A2 occurs first, approximately .03 to .06 seconds before P2, and reflects the shorter ejection time of the left ventricle. Some normal physiological splitting of S2 can be appreciated with inspiration which reflects the augmented right ventricle flow that occurs with this phase of respiration.

25

In addition to these heart sounds, two low frequency diastolic sounds can sometimes be heard in normal individuals

S3 is the first diastolic heart sound occurring 0.12 to 0.20 seconds after the passive ventricular filling stage is completed. It occurs just after the T wave on ECG and is caused by passive filling of the ventricles, vibrating of the AV valves, and their supporting structures. This sounds occurs after S2 heart sound.

S4 is sound due to blood turbulence in atrial systole. If the patient has any known cardiac anomalies, this sound would be considered abnormal.

left apex and the tricuspid valve is best heard at the fourth intercostal space left sternal border. Abnormal heart sounds can be caused by a number of different abnormalities but the most common are due to valvular stenosis or regurgitations.

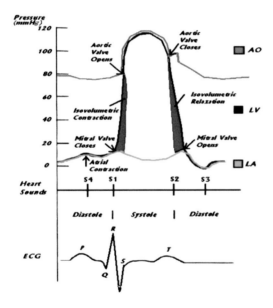

Wigger's Diagram

Listening to heart sounds is called auscultation and is usually performed by a stethoscope. The heart valves are best heard in certain areas on the chest due to the location of the valves. The aortic valve is best heard at the second intercostal space on the right sternal border (2RIS). The pulmonic valve is best heard at the 2LIS, second intercostal space left sternal border. The mitral valve is best heard at the

ANATOMY AND PHYSIOLOGY QUIZ

1. Rapid depolarization correlates with this ECG waveform:
   a. S wave
   b. T wave
   c. P wave
   d. QRS complex

2. What phase of the cardiac cycle demonstrates four valve closure, the ventricles are contracting and pressure is increasing?
   a. Isovolumetric relaxation
   b. Ventricular systole
   c. Isovolumetric contraction
   d. Ventricular diastole

3. The area of the heart where the coronary sulcus meets the interventricular sulcus is called the:
   a. apex
   b. crux
   c. coronary sinus
   d. AV groove

4. The inner surface of the heart wall is the:
   a. myocardium
   b. epicardium
   c. visceral layer
   d. endocardium

5. Which of the heart wall layers is responsible for the heart's ability to contract?
   a. parietal pericardium
   b. myocardium
   c. epicardium
   d. endocardium

6. The left ventricular outflow tract ends at the level of the:
   a. aortic annulus
   b. left ventricle
   c. papillary muscles
   d. chordae tendineae

7. The most anterior chamber of the heart is the:
   a. left ventricle
   b. left atrium
   c. right ventricle
   d. right atrium

8. What structure in the right ventricle extends from the lower interventricular septum to the anterior wall where it joins the papillary muscle?
   a. chordae tendineae
   b. tricuspid valve
   c. moderator band
   d. trabeculations

9. The right ventricular outflow tract is also referred to as the:
   a. conus arteriosus
   b. crista supraventricularis
   c. infundibulum
   d. b and d
   e. a and c

10. What are the normal number of pulmonary veins?
    a. 6
    b. 2
    c. 3
    d. 4 to 5

11. Where are the pectinate muscles located in left atrium?
    a. whole left atrium
    b. pulmonary veins
    c. posterior left atrial wall
    d. left atrial appendage

12. The cardiac structure that forms the right lateral cardiac border is the:
    a. left ventricle
    b. right ventricle
    c. right atrium
    d. left atrium

13. Which three structures empty blood into the right atrium?
    a. IVC, SVC, coronary sinus
    b. coronary sinus, IVC, coronary arteries
    c. IVC, SVC, aorta
    d. aorta, pulmonary veins, coronary sinus

14. The Eustachian valve is located in the:
    a. SVC
    b. IVC
    c. coronary sinus
    d. aorta

15. S1 heart sound correlates with this waveform on the ECG?
    a. S wave
    b. T wave
    c. P wave
    d. QRS complex

16. Normal pericardial fluid lies between which two pericardial layers?
    a. fibrous and serous
    b. myocardium and epicardium
    c. visceral and parietal
    d. endocardium and myocardium

17. The support structures at the end of each of the aortic valve cusps are called the:
    a. Lambl's excrescences
    b. Arantius's nodules
    c. sinuses of Valsalva
    d. AV nodes

18. The largest of the tricuspid valve leaflets is the:
    a. posterior
    b. inferior
    c. anterior
    d. septal

19. Which coronary artery feeds the right atrium, right ventricle and inferior wall of the left ventricle?
    a. left circumflex
    b. coronary sinus
    c. right coronary artery
    d. left anterior descending

20. What structure is continuous with the posterior aortic root wall?
    a. interventricular septum
    b. papillary muscle
    c. posterolateral mitral leaflet
    d. anteromedial mitral leaflet

21. The origin of both the aorta and the pulmonary artery is the:
    a. embryonic truncus arteriosus
    b. ligamentum venosum
    c. sinuses of Valsalva
    d. conus aorticus

22. Which one of the following is NOT usually a direct branch off of the aortic arch?
    a. left common carotid artery
    b. left subclavian artery
    c. brachiocephalic
    d. innominate
    e. right common carotid artery

23. Isovolumetric relaxation occurs:
    a. Just after the P wave
    b. Midway through the QRS
    c. Just after the T wave
    d. Just after aortic valve opening

24. Aortic valve opening occurs with this waveform on the ECG?
    a. U wave
    b. T wave
    c. P wave
    d. QRS complex

25. The great cardiac vein anastomoses with the:
    a. aortic arch
    b. right coronary artery
    c. oblique vein of Marshal
    d. oblique vein of Galen

26. The second heart sound is made by the:
    a. opening of the mitral valve
    b. closing of the aortic valve
    c. closing of the mitral valve
    d. opening of the aortic valve

27. What percentage of blood does atrial contraction contribute to left ventricular filling?
    a. 15-30%
    b. 50-60%
    c. 100%
    d. 0%

28. The primary pacemaker in the heart is the:
    a. AV node
    b. Purkinje fibers
    c. sino-atrial node
    d. bundle of His

29. The T wave on the EKG represents:
    a. atrial depolarization
    b. ventricular contraction
    c. atrial repolarization
    d. ventricular repolarization

30. The amount of blood pumped out of the aorta with every heart beat is referred to as:
    a. stroke volume
    b. cardiac output
    c. ejection fraction
    d. cardiac index

31. Identify which location demonstrates aortic valve closure on the pressure waveform seen below?
    a. 1
    b. 2
    c. 3
    d. 4

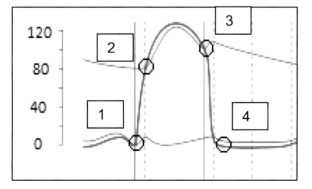

32. The relationship between length and tension is determined by:
    a. Frank Starling law
    b. Poiseuille's law
    c. Bernoulli equation
    d. Reynolds number

33. The coronary arteries arise from this area of the aorta:
    a. aortic arch
    b. sinotubular junction
    c. sinus of Valsalva
    d. descending aorta

34. Identify which location demonstrates ventricular systole?
    a. 1
    b. 2

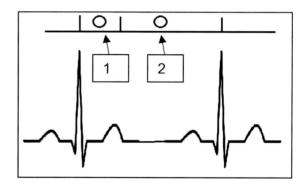

35. Approximately what percentage of blood filling occurs in the left ventricle during early diastolic filling?
    a. 15%
    b. 50%
    c. 70%
    d. 100%

36. Label the following events at the indicated circles on the ECG:

Mitral valve closure
Ventricular repolarization
Aortic valve opening
Atrial systole

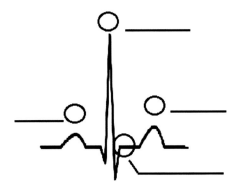

37. What small branches arise from the RCA?
    a. Septal perforators
    b. Obtuse marginals
    c. Acute marginals
    d. Diagonal

38. The most anterior structure of the heart is the?
    a. left atrium
    b. right atrium
    c. left ventricle
    d. right ventricle

39. The coronary arteries mainly perfuse during this part of the cardiac cycle?
    a. Systole
    b. Diastole

40. What occurs during the holding phase of the Valsalva maneuver?
    a. Increase venous return
    b. Increase cardiac output
    c. Decrease venous return
    d. Decrease cardiac contraction

41. Which of the two atrioventricular valves sit more apically in the heart?
    a. Mitral
    b. Tricuspid
    c. Pulmonic
    d. Aortic

42. The ability of a myocardial cell to spontaneous depolarize is called:
    a. Conductivity
    b. Automaticity
    c. Excitability
    d. Contractility

43. What opens and closes the valves in the heart?
    a. Pressure changes
    b. Electrical stimulation
    c. Muscles
    d. Brain stimulation

44. Which phase of diastole does not occur in patients with atrial fibrillation:
    a. Rapid filling
    b. Slow filling
    c. Diastasis
    d. Atrial systole

GULFCOAST
ULTRASOUND
INSTITUTE INC

Section 2:

Technique

Section 2: TECHNIQUE

Objectives

Upon completion of this module you should be able to:
- Optimize equipment controls
- Recognize commonly seen technical artifacts
- Integrate standardized imaging views to perform a two-dimensional cardiac ultrasound exam
- Identify regional wall segments
- Recognize normal M-mode patterns
- Utilize optimal scanning views and appropriate interrogation angles for performing Doppler studies
- Compare benefits of using contrast agents to standard 2D imaging
- State how to apply the use of provocative maneuvers in echocardiography
- State the routine imaging planes used for transesophageal echocardiography
- Outline the basic CPR protocols

TECHNIQUE

USE OF EQUIPMENT CONTROLS

The **depth** control affects several parameters relating to the ultrasound image. For adult echocardiography it is recommended to begin with a standard imaging depth of approximately 15 to 16 cm for a parasternal long axis (PLAX) view which allows for quick recognition of enlarged chambers or overall cardiomegaly. However, remember that the optimum depth is directly dependent on the size of the patient and transducer position.

When the area being imaged is larger, a greater depth is required. Make sure to allow for some visualization of structures beyond the pericardium to exclude pericardial or pleural effusion. The depth can then be readjusted to fill the screen with the pertinent cardiac anatomy. Increasing the depth results in a decrease in the pulse repetition frequency since it will take longer for the pulse to travel back and forth from the transducer. The effect on frame rate should be minimal. When performing pulsed wave Doppler, the PRF is important in that it determines the Nyquist Limit. Pay close attention to the depth if you are performing PW Doppler and the waveform is aliasing.

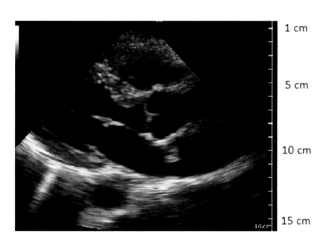

1 cm

5 cm

10 cm

15 cm

Sample of Depth of Image

The **amplification** of the sound is controlled by the gain or DGC/TGC (depth or time gain compensation). If the whole image is too dark or too bright, the overall gain controls should be used.

DGC/TGC controls can also selectively adjust the amplification or brightness of the image in specific areas or regions based upon depth. This is typically controlled by the use of slide pods or toggle switches associated with these regions of the ultrasound image.

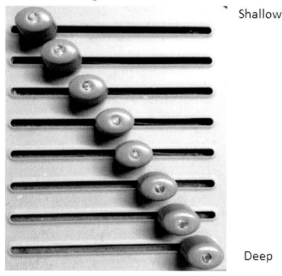

Shallow

Deep

Sample of TGC keys on ultrasound system

Near and far field gain controls may also be used to selectively adjust those areas respectively. Rotary knobs may also be used for these functions and for the overall gain.

Transmit power is the voltage which is applied to the transducer itself. This controls the intensity of the sound beam. Transmit power should be kept at lower settings following the *"ALARA"* principle; *As Low As Reasonably Achievable* since it may be associated with some biological effects.

The **focal zone** is the region where the best resolution can be obtained. Most systems allow the operator to adjust or move the focal zones on a real time image. Altering the focal zone allows for the beam to be collimated for a specific area of the image. Beyond the focal zone the beam diverges and therefore it should be set at or just below the main structure or area of interest in your field of view. Setting the focal zone too anterior to the structure of interest places it in the divergent portion of the beam which reduces its effectiveness. For example, from an apical four chamber view when interrogating the apex, it should be set in the near field and when interrogating the mitral valve, the focus should be set more in the far field. The operator can add multiple focal zones but this will lower the frame rate which may not be desirable.

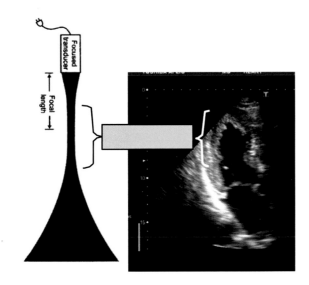

Focal Zone demonstrating Apex in focal zone but MV & LA is in divergent portion of beam profile

Sector Width of the transducer is also important. Widening the sector width will cause a decrease in the frame rate. Always keep the sector width as narrow as possible to maintain higher frame rates.

Dynamic range in gray scale imaging is the smallest to largest group of intensities which produce a shade of gray on the monitor. Most equipment has a larger dynamic range than the human eye can perceive. The greater the dynamic range, the more potential gray scale shades. If the dynamic range is reduced, the shades of gray are decreased and the image contrast increases which may improve edge detection of the endocardium and make the chambers look more cystic. Be careful though not to enhance the chambers with too much contrast or "blood pools" too black as it may exclude isoechoic or low level thrombus which might otherwise be detected.

Pre-processing allows for the altering or changing of the signal before the image is frozen while post processing alters the signal afterwards. Pre and Post processing will sometimes help to enhance an image that is technically limited. *"Write"* and *"Read"* zoom features are an example of *Pre & Post* processing functions respectively. *"Write"* zoom works on a live image and a *"Read"* zoom works on a frozen image.

The **Doppler angle** in cardiac, as well as in all ultrasound applications, is optimum when it is at zero degrees to flow or parallel to flow. The incident angle should be no greater than 20^0 to flow when performing cardiac Doppler. Doppler angles greater than 20^0 result in large calculation errors. The best rule to consider when performing any type of Doppler exam is, the lower the angle of incidence to flow, the better the returning or reflected signal. Angle correction controls allow for the exact measurement of the angle of incidence relative to the direction of flow. Angle correction controls are typically not utilized for cardiac Doppler since the Doppler views used are typically between $0°$ and $20°$ and the difference in the cosine value of $0°$ to $20°$ is very minimal. *See the following Cosine table.*

Cosines for Various Angles	
Angle A (Degrees)	cos A
0	1.00
5	0.996
10	0.98
15	0.97
20	0.94
25	0.91
30	0.87
35	0.82
40	0.77
45	0.71
50	0.64
55	0.57
60	0.50
65	0.42
70	0.34
75	0.26
80	0.17
85	0.09
90	0.00

Filters are electronic devices used to separate or remove certain components of a complex waveform. There are several types of filters used with Doppler instruments such as band pass, high pass, and low pass filters. High pass filters permit the frequencies above which the filter is tuned to be transmitted, while eliminating frequencies below this point. The opposite is true for low pass filters. The theory behind the band pass filter is to attenuate frequencies lying outside the band pass and transmitting those within the band pass. The pass band is the portion of the frequency bandwidth that is allowed to pass through a filter. The portion of the frequency bandwidth that is removed is called the stop band.

The **sample volume or sample gate** is used for pulsed Doppler modalities. The sample gate or range gate is site specific and gives flow information specific to the area or the vessel that it is placed. The term used to describe this function is sometimes referred to as range resolution. The gate length may be increased or decreased to allow for a larger or smaller sampling area. The range of the sample gate is usually 1-20 mm. A longer gate usually improves the signal to noise ratio. Sample gate or sample volume width is

always equal to the beam width at the site of the sample volume.

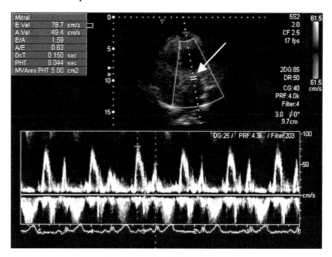

Sample Gate/Volume

Zero shift or baseline controls allow for the baseline to be moved up or down depending on the Doppler signal, direction of the signal, and signal velocity. If a Doppler signal is cut off or aliases, the baseline can be adjusted to try to include the entire spectral signal. When the Doppler signal continues to cut off after the zero baseline is adjusted as much as possible, the pulse repetition frequency or PRF can be increased. When this fails to include the entire Doppler signal on the spectral tracing, continuous wave Doppler should be implemented to resolve the aliased signal.

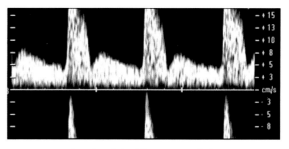

Baseline needs to be shifted down to avoid aliasing

37

Pulse repetition frequency or PRF may be referred to as velocity range or scale. The pulse repetition frequency is the number of pulses per second or other specified unit of time. When the pulse repetition frequency is increased, higher velocity signals can be detected. When the pulse repetition frequency is decreased the velocity range is decreased improving sensitivity to slower flow. PRF is also dependent upon depth of the image. Nyquist limit is equal to ½ of the PRF.

Spectral analysis is the breaking up of the parts of a complex wave. These parts are spread out in the order of their frequencies. With the use of FFT or Fast Fourier Transformer, the Doppler spectrum is derived from the various frequencies of the returning signals. This technique can demonstrate frequency, amplitude, and spectral broadening that results from a wide range of Doppler shifted frequencies.

On the spectral display, time is displayed on the horizontal axis corresponding to changes in the cardiac cycle and frequency shifts towards (+) or away (-) from the transducer are displayed above or below the zero baseline respectively. Although the system is detecting frequency shifts, most newer systems display the calculated velocities on the vertical axis assuming the incident angle was 0° to 20° and thus using a cosine value of one.

The brightness of the gray scale spectrum analysis represents the number of events at that Doppler shifted frequency. Spectral broadening refers to the range of frequencies at any moment in time and is relative to the vertical axis of the spectrum analysis. A thicker waveform would indicate spectral broadening.

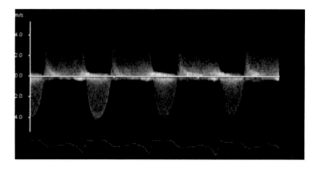

Spectral Display

The **resonant frequency** of a transducer is its operating frequency. The propagation speed of the transducer material and the thickness of the transducer element determine its operating frequency. Most adult echocardiography is performed with transducer frequencies of 2.0 to 5.0 MHz. The higher the frequency of the transducer the better the resolution, but penetration is decreased. Broad bandwidth or multi-frequency transducers allow a variety of both selectable imaging and Doppler frequencies for optimal resolution and penetration.

There are several types of transducers utilized in ultrasound imaging. A commonly used transducer in adult echocardiography is a **sector phased array** transducer. This type of transducer has several elements in the transducer head. Voltage pulses are applied to all of the elements, but at small time differences which allows the beam to be shaped and steered. Phased array transducers are quiet, lightweight and have more flexibility of beam angulation, field of depth, and sector width.

Additionally, phased array transducers allow for simultaneous B & W imaging and the use of other modalities such as m-mode, pulsed Doppler, and color flow imaging. These transducers also offer continuous wave (CW) Doppler but the imaging function is updated between CW Doppler acquisition and is operator selectable on most systems. A phased array transducer can use dynamic focusing in the receiver, and fixed, but detectable focusing in the transmitter.

The main disadvantage of phased array transducers is the increased side lobe intensity, but many manufacturers have overcome this artifact with apodization or other noise reducing techniques. Some phased array transducers use a lens or curvature to focus the elevational plane which limits focusing in the thickness dimension. Digital beam formation and dynamic aperture and dynamic frequency techniques have improved this limitation in phased array transducers. Phased array transducers produce a sector shaped image display.

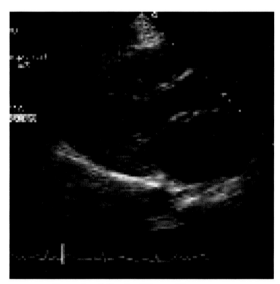

Sample of Sector Shaped Image

Mechanical transducers obtain images by either rapidly oscillating one crystal in an arc or rotating multiple crystals mechanically. These transducers are sometimes lower in cost and in certain instances, have better resolution. There are numerous disadvantages for these transducers for cardiac applications such as: the larger size, increased maintenance of the transducer due to the mechanical parts, the Doppler shift created by the movement of the crystal that results in limitations for Doppler and color flow imaging, and the vibrations produced by the transducer.

Annular array transducers contain multiple elements arranged in a ring. This is a hybrid of mechanical and array technology. Advantages of these transducers are: good penetration, focusing capabilities, uniform image sharpness, increased lateral resolution, and they have the thinnest tomographic image slices. The disadvantage is the mechanical mechanism limits its usefulness for rapidly moving cardiac structures and multi-tasking cardiac applications. Mechanical and annular array transducers aren't offered with current systems, however they may still be in use by facilities that have older or used equipment in the echo lab.

Matrix array transducers are electronically steered and have on average 2,000 to 3,000 elements. Phasing the large number of elements arranged in a matrix enables the acquisition of several scan planes simultaneously. For instance, both the parasternal long and short-axis or apical 4 chamber and 2 chamber 2D scan planes of the heart can be shown. In addition, it allows an individual scan plane to be swept or rotated through a 3 dimensional volume of tissue.

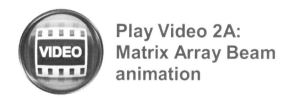

Play Video 2A:
Matrix Array Beam
animation

The matrix array transducers have a slightly larger footprint and overall size and they are more expensive to purchase and maintain under service contract. However, in addition to their multiplane view and 3D applications, most of the matrix array transducers have some 4D capabilities too which offer both current and future advantages for cardiac applications.

RECOGNITION OF TECHNICAL ARTIFACTS

Artifacts in ultrasound are anything on the picture or display which does not belong to the structures being imaged and are not real.

Reverberation artifacts are high-amplitude, linear artifacts that result from two strong specular reflectors. These create a back and forth reflection of the ultrasound before it can return to the transducer creating a redundant malposition series of reflectors going in different directions from the main sound beam. This results in reflectors being placed on areas in the wrong location on the image. Multiple reflectors may be noted in different locations on the image.

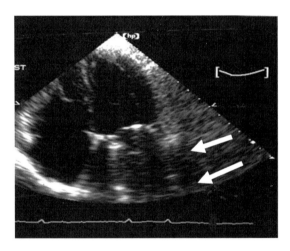

Reverberation Artifact from Mechanical Valve

Mirror images are often seen in cardiac imaging. Mirror images are seen when objects which are on one side of a strong reflector are also noted on the other side.

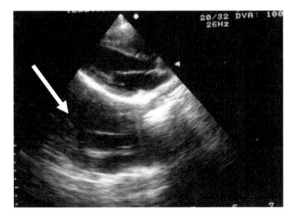

Mirror Image Artifact

Side lobe artifacts are caused by the acoustic energy emitted by the transducer going in different directions from the main sound beam. This results in reflectors being placed on areas in the wrong location on the image. Multiple reflectors may be noted in different locations on the image.

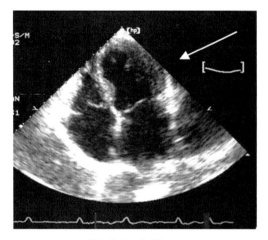

Side Lobe Artifact
(potentially false appearance of Apical Clot)

Acoustic shadowing may occur as a result of the sound beam encountering dense objects such as bone or calcifications in the body. These structures impede the sound causing attenuation that results in an acoustic shadow or drop out effect.

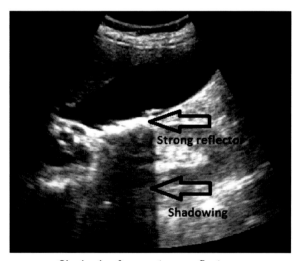

Shadowing from a strong reflector

Aliasing of the color signal occurs when the flow exceeds the Nyquist limit. Color flow Doppler aliasing occurs at lower

40

velocities than conventional pulsed Doppler. Color Doppler aliasing is seen as one color folding over into the opposite color. Once aliasing patterns are recognized however, this artifact does not pose a significant problem and can help with the detection of certain cardiac anomalies. Aliasing alone is not a diagnostic criterion to indicate pathology.

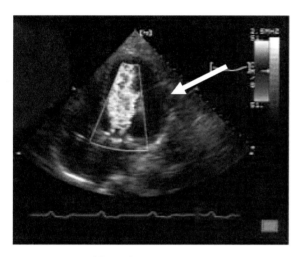

Aliasing of Color Signal with Mitral Stenosis

Wall motion of the heart can produce signals that are stronger than the signals being produced by the red blood cells, resulting in an artifact. Some of this can be eliminated with the use of reject and wall filters. Color flow imaging may not be as sensitive as conventional pulsed Doppler causing weak signals to be missed. When the Color gain is increased color noise can be created. Color noise appears as a speckling of color that can occur inside or outside of the structure being evaluated.

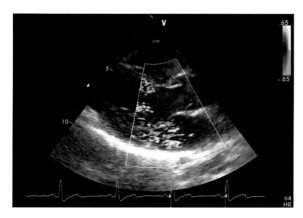

Color Speckling or Noise

Temporal ambiguity may result when lower frame rates are utilized for color flow Doppler. Lower frame rates are used with color due to the increased time it takes to create a color flow image. The size of the sector can impact frame rate. A narrower, color sector or ROI (region of interest) box allows for faster frame rates and a wider sector or color ROI box decreases or slows frame rate.

Ghosting is an artifact seen with black and white imaging and color flow imaging. It is the brief appearance of large patterns of gray noise or color displayed over anatomic structures and are not related to any associated flow patterns. Ghosting is a result of strong moving reflectors and is commonly seen in patients with prosthetic heart valves.

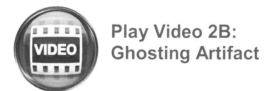 Play Video 2B: Ghosting Artifact

RECOGNITION OF SETUP ERRORS

All ultrasound system manufacturers offer programmable PRE SETS for a wide variety of exam modalities. This configures the initial set-up of the system for the type of study to be performed and adjusts many system parameters and controls to the preferred operation standards for that facility and for that ultrasound examination. For instance, it can select the appropriate transducer and initial imaging depth, monitor and probe orientation, focus location, gray scale settings and factory or programmable measurement and calculation packages for cardiac vs other examinations or for 2D vs. Doppler applications.

Easy recognition of set up errors would be by the image orientation, depth settings,

41

annotation or labeling selections, body icons or automated protocols or the measurement and/or calculation package that is recalled when activated. Most systems also display somewhere on the monitor which PRE SET has been selected and make it easy to recognize if any of the parameters appear incorrect.

Activating the appropriate PRE SET will change the system configuration without requiring re-inputting the patient information in most cases or requiring the operator to navigate all the necessary changes to system parameters independently. Some system manufacturers ask the operator to select the type of exam to be performed when inputting the patient ID information making this step quite simple and helping to avoid set-up errors.

TWO-DIMENSIONAL STUDY

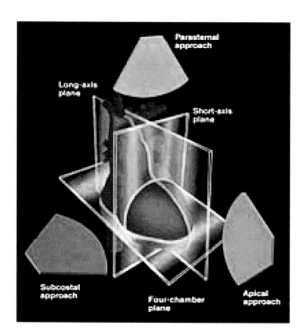

The basic echocardiogram usually includes four scan planes. The parasternal position is usually the starting point. The transducer is optimally placed in the 3rd to 4th intercostal rib space and as close to the sternum as possible. This allows for the most accuracy when obtaining measurements. Variations of this position

can be used to show pertinent cardiac anatomy and abnormalities.

In the **parasternal** position the heart can be viewed in numerous scan planes. The standard planes are the parasternal long and short axis views. The **long axis** view images the heart in a lengthwise or longitudinal plane. With the PLA view, the transducer is placed in the 4LIS with the indicator marker pointing towards the right shoulder. The structures usually noted in this view are the right ventricle, and right ventricle wall which is the most anterior structure. Below the right ventricle lies the interventricular septum, left ventricle, and the infero-lateral, formerly posterior wall.

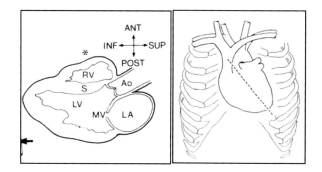

Parasternal Long Axis view diagram & orientation

If the transducer is moved inferiorly and laterally the apex may be seen. Also at the top of the screen is the right ventricular outflow tract which is merely an extension of the right ventricle. Below this is the aortic root and valve, left atrium and mitral valve. The descending aorta is seen in cross-section posterior to the left atrium and is seen as a circle. The coronary sinus may also be noted between the left atrium and mitral valve.

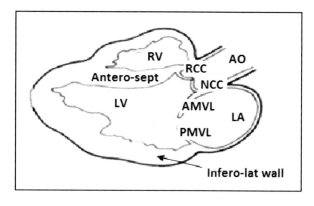

Anatomy of the PLAX view

42

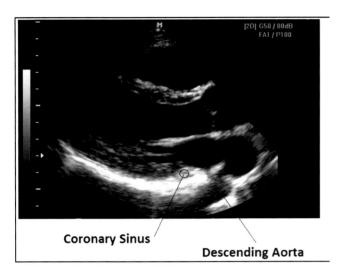

Anatomy of Coronary Sinus and DA

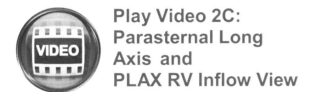

Play Video 2C:
Parasternal Long Axis and
PLAX RV Inflow View

If the transducer is angled medially and slightly inferiorly (towards the patients right hip) the right ventricle inflow region and tricuspid valve may be seen. In this view you can see the right atrium, the ostium of the coronary sinus and IVC in some patients and the right ventricle. Typically, from this view you will see the anterior tricuspid valve leaflet and the septal tricuspid valve leaflet but depending on the angle it may be the posterior leaflet instead of the septal leaflet.

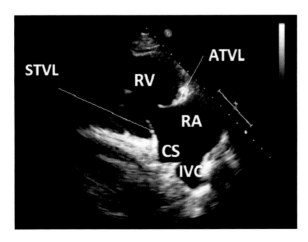

Anatomy of RVIT view

Another less commonly used parasternal view is the Right Ventricle Outflow View. This view is obtained by angling the scan plane from the PLAX superiorly and medially to visualize the RVOT, PV and proximal pulmonary artery. This window is also used with color flow imaging and Doppler modalities to assess flow across the pulmonic valve and is good for assessing pulmonic stenosis or regurgitation. It is less common because of varying or lower degrees of success in obtaining this view.

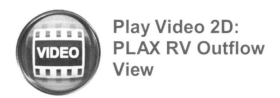

Play Video 2D:
PLAX RV Outflow View

Rotating the transducer 90 degrees clockwise from the PLAX view results in a **short axis** or cross-sectional view of the heart.

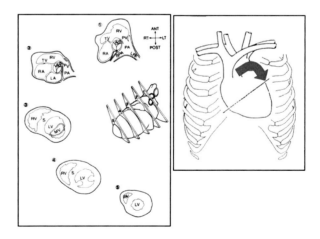

Parasternal Short Axis View diagram & orientation

43

Tilting the transducer superiorly and inferiorly, various cardiac structures can be displayed according to the planes in the previous diagram. This is called the Parasternal short-axis view at the level of the aortic valve. Angling the transducer superiorly and towards the patient's right shoulder the right atrium, right ventricular outflow tract, tricuspid valve, aortic valve, left atrium, pulmonic valve, and pulmonary artery may be seen. Also, the left atrial appendage may be visualized in the PSAX of the aortic valve. If the transducer is angled beyond the AV level or more superiorly, the aortic root or proximal ascending aorta, main pulmonary artery and right & left pulmonary artery branches may be demonstrated in some patients.

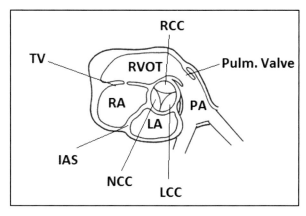

Anatomy of PSAX view at Aortic Level

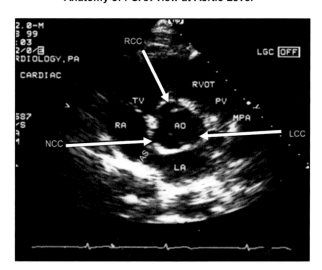

Image of PSAX view at Aortic Level

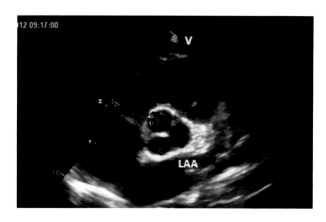

Image of the left atrial appendage from a PSAX Aortic Level View

When the transducer is angled from the patient's right shoulder towards the patients left hip other cardiac structures will be seen. Next to come into view is the mitral valve known as the parasternal short axis view at the mitral valve level. The anterior and posterior mitral valve leaflets are seen along with the right ventricle and basilar level of the left ventricle.

As the angulation continues towards the left hip the chordae tendineae and papillary muscles will be seen along with the heart walls. This view is known as the parasternal short axis at the level of the LV/Papillary. In a clockwise fashion starting at approximately 10 or 11 o'clock the walls of the heart seen are the interventricular septum (divided into two segments: inferoseptum and anteroseptum), the anterior wall, the lateral wall (divided into two segments: anterolateral & inferolateral) and the inferior wall (see following diagram). The right ventricle walls may also be seen.

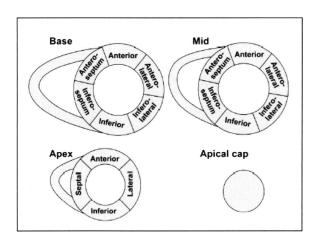

Nomenclature for Labeling LV wall segments based upon ASE guidelines

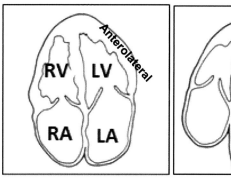

Apical Four Chamber & Apical Five Chamber View

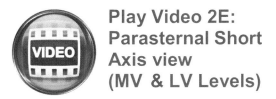

Play Video 2E:
Parasternal Short Axis view
(MV & LV Levels)

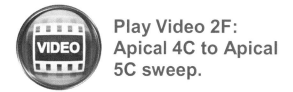

Play Video 2F:
Apical 4C to Apical 5C sweep.

The **apical transducer** position may be found by locating the patients PMI or point of maximal impulse of the heart with the indicator marker pointing to about 3 o'clock. This is usually near or below the left breast. Thinner patients may have lower more lateral transducer positions while heavier patients tend to have higher more medial positions. Also, as patients age their apex seems to "migrate" toward a higher position in the axillary plane due to less elasticity of the supporting structures. The net result is the heart may have more of a horizontal axis in the chest rather than a diagonal axis from right shoulder to left hip.

To obtain the apical 4 chamber view the transducer is placed at the PMI and rotated until the four chambers of the heart are seen. On this view both atria and ventricles are seen, as well as the apex, left ventricle lateral wall, interventricular septum, right ventricle lateral wall, and interatrial septum. If the transducer is angled superiorly the aorta will be viewed as well as the left ventricular outflow tract. When the addition of the aorta and LVOT are displayed this apical window is referred to as the apical 5 chamber view.

When the transducer is rotated 45 degrees counter clock-wise from the apical 4C view or to the left, the **apical two chamber** view is obtained. This allows visualization of the left ventricle, left atrium, mitral valve, inferior and anterior walls of the heart. The rotation is complete when the RV disappears from view and the coronary sinus is visualized as a round or ovoid structure on the left side of the monitor, lateral to and sometimes slightly posterior to the mitral annulus. The left atrial appendage may also be visualized in the apical two chamber image.

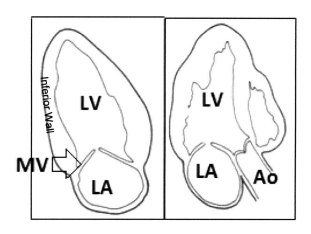

Apical Two & Apical Three Chamber View

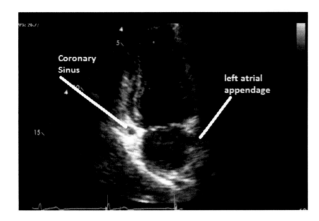

**Image of Coronary Sinus and Left Atrial Appendage
From an Apical Two Chamber Image**

**Play Video 2G:
Apical 2C rotate to
Apical 3C view**

Extending the counter clockwise rotation an additional 30-45 degrees from the apical 2 Chamber view with a slight superior angulation produces the **apical long axis or apical 3 chamber** view of the heart. This view demonstrates the left ventricle, left atrium, aorta, left ventricular outflow tract, the inferolateral and anteroseptum heart walls. These are the same structures that were visualized from the parasternal long axis view but positioned from the apex which is now at the top of the screen and which presents a parallel direction rather than perpendicular direction to flow. Therefore, this view is more commonly used as an alternative or complementary view to the Apical 5 chamber view to interrogate the LVOT, aortic valve, proximal aorta, and the mitral apparatus with Doppler and color flow imaging modalities.

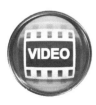

**Play video 2H:
Apical 3 Chamber or
Apical Long Axis
View**

If the transducer is placed in the xyphoid process region and angled superiorly and to the patient's left, the **subcostal view** of the heart is obtained. The indicator marker in this view is pointing to 3 o'clock. The four chambers of the heart and variations of the long and short axis views may be obtained from this position. This view uses the left lobe of the liver as a window to look at the heart. The 4 chamber subcostal view includes the right ventricle, tricuspid valve, right atrium, interventricular septum, interatrial septum, left ventricle, left atrium, and mitral valve. Elevating the scan plane anteriorly reveals the aortic valve and proximal aortic root and with slightly further elevation the RVOT and main pulmonary artery and the right and left branches and pulmonic valve may be seen on this view.

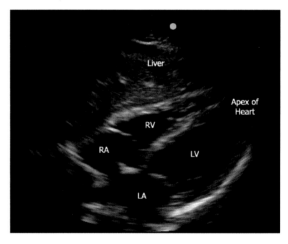

4-Chamber Subcostal View

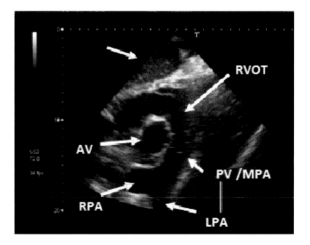

Subcoastal view of main PA, PV, and RPA & LPA

When the transducer is rotated counter clockwise and angled slightly towards the patients right, the inferior vena cava and hepatic veins may be seen. The abdominal aorta can also be imaged when the transducer is angled inferior from the heart and slightly left of the midline. This probe orientation also allows for cross-sectional imaging of the LV as the beam is swept from the base of the LV to the apex or from the patient's midline towards the patient's left axilla.

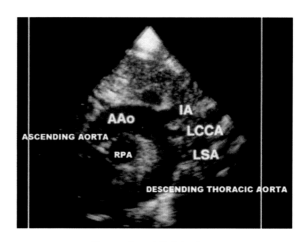

Suprasternal Notch view

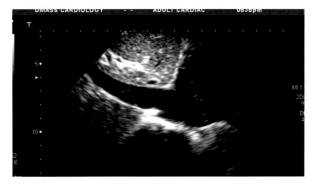

Subcostal View of IVC

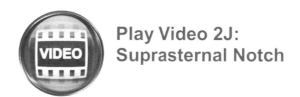

Play Video 2J:
Suprasternal Notch

The **suprasternal view** is obtained by locating the transducer in the suprasternal notch and angling the transducer inferiorly.

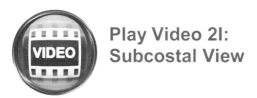

Play Video 2I:
Subcostal View

Depending on transducer rotation, the ascending aorta, descending aorta, aortic arch, and vessels off the arch can be seen. The brachiocephalic artery or innominate artery typically arises from the right side of the aortic arch. The left common carotid artery, and left subclavian artery arise from the left side of the aortic arch. The right pulmonary artery can be seen on end inferior to the arch.

VENTRICULAR WALL SEGMENTS

American Society of Echocardiography recommends the division of the left ventricle into seventeen segments at the basal, mid, and apical levels. The parasternal long axis view demonstrates the basal and mid inferolateral and anteroseptal walls. The apical inferolateral and anteroseptal walls, as well as the apical cap, are seen from the apical three-chamber view.

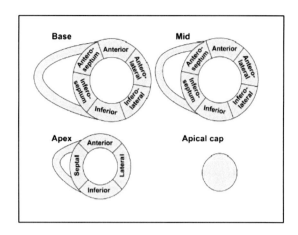

PSAX Wall Segments

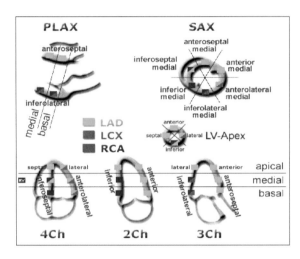

ASE Recommended Wall Segments

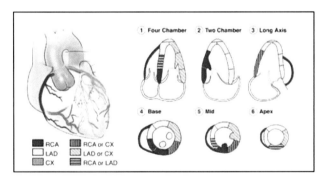

Coronary Distribution

The short axis view of the heart demonstrates all basal, mid and apical walls at their respective tomographic imaging level.

The true apical cap is rarely seen from the parasternal approach even with extreme apical angulation.

48

M-mode Patterns

M-mode functions may also be used when performing echocardiography. M-mode stands for motion mode. The signals are generated just like the B-mode signals but are isolated to a single line of information and have much better temporal resolution (1 to 3 μsec.) relative to movement of various cardiac structures.

M-mode uses a single beam or single line of sight so only one line of information is recorded at a time. This means that wherever the M-line or cursor is placed in the heart, that area alone is being evaluated. Each part of the heart is depicted by a different M-mode configuration. The M-mode tracings are placed on a calibrated grid, which allows for timing of cardiac events and measurement of structures; the y-axis of the display is depth and the x-axis is time. The parasternal long and short axis views are the usual planes in which an M-mode exam may be performed. When the m-line or cursor is placed through a particular section of the heart, a single plane recording of the area is obtained. M-mode is helpful since it records movement and depth of structures. It samples at a rate of 1800 frames per second rather than the 30 or so that is done with 2-dimensional imaging. This allows for acquisition of cardiac movements too fast for the human eye to otherwise detect.

M-Mode of the Aortic Valve

When the cursor or M-line is placed through the aorta at the valve level, the right ventricular outflow tract, aortic root, valve, and left atrium are displayed. In systole the valve forms a box-like structure and in diastole it appears as a long, thin line that should be seen in the middle of the root. Premature closure of the aortic valve tracing on M-mode would appear as a small triangular shape and could suggest possible subvalvular obstruction. The left atrium is located posterior to the aortic root and is normally the same size or slightly larger than

the aortic root. The normal aortic root to left atrium ratio is 1:1.3.

Fine fluttering of the aortic cusps may be noted on the M-mode tracing of the valve and usually reflects good cardiac output. The aortic root wall motion depends on left atrial filling. Exaggerated root motion may be seen when there is increased left atrial filling and emptying, as in cases of mitral regurgitation. Decreased aortic root wall motion is noted in low cardiac output states when the left atrial filling and emptying is decreased.

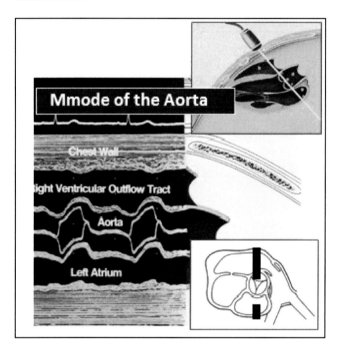

Aortic Valve M-mode tracing

The anterior aortic root wall is continuous with the interventricular septum and the posterior aortic root wall is continuous with the anterior mitral valve leaflet. The descending aorta may be seen as an echo-free structure beneath the left atrium.

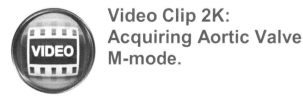

Video Clip 2K: Acquiring Aortic Valve M-mode.

M-Mode of the Mitral Valve

When the cursor is moved to the tips of the mitral valve leaflets a tracing of the mitral valve and leaflet motion is obtained. The interventricular septum is located anterior to the anterior mitral leaflet while the infero-lateral wall lies posterior to the posterior mitral valve leaflet. The right ventricle is also seen anterior to the interventricular septum. The mitral tracing has an "M" configuration which corresponds to the two phases of diastole. When the mitral valve is closed both leaflets should form a line. This line called the line of closure is seen during systole. When the valve is open the "M" configuration begins. The normal posterior leaflet forms a mirror image to the anterior leaflet.

The end of systole or onset of diastole on the valve tracing is called the D point. When the valve is at its maximum leaflet separation in early diastole the first peak of the "M" configuration is the E point. The DE points represent the early or rapid filling phase of diastole. The valve begins to drift shut and is called the F point. This occurs because the pressure is equalizing between the left atria and left ventricle and is called diastasis or EF slope. Next an electrical stimulus causes atrial systole or atrial contraction resulting in 20-30% more blood to be ejected through the valve and into the left ventricle.

This second spike that appears on the "M" tracing is called the A point which is the second phase of diastole and corresponds to the late filling from atrial systole. When the valve finally closes at the end of diastole it is called the C point. If a bump or notch is noted between the A and C points it may be called a "B" bump or notch or an A-C shoulder. This may be an indication of elevated left ventricular end diastolic pressure.

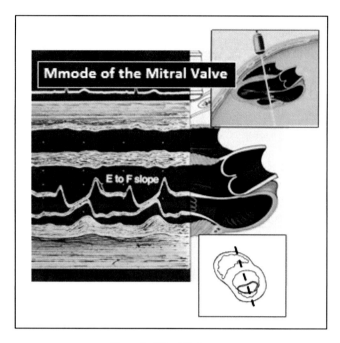

M-mode Mitral Valve

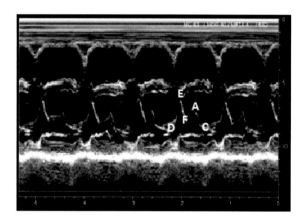

M-mode Mitral Valve tracing

The distance between the E point and the interventricular septum is called the EPSS or E point to septal separation. An increased EPSS may indicate left ventricular dilatation or systolic dysfunction. An EPSS > 2cm suggests <50% ejection fraction. However, false positive results can occur with mitral stenosis and aortic insufficiency. These conditions can restrict motion of the anterior mitral valve leaflet causing an exaggerated EPSS in an otherwise normal size and functioning left ventricle. On the image below notice how the aortic insufficiency jet is hitting the anterior mitral valve leaflet.

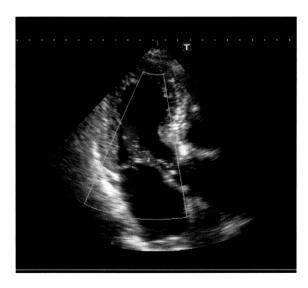

Aortic insufficiency Jet restricting motion of ALMV

M-Mode of the Left Ventricle

When the cursor is placed just past the mitral leaflet tips the right ventricle anterior wall, right ventricle, interventricular septum, left ventricle, inferolateral wall (previously called the posterior wall) and pericardium are viewed. These structures' size, motion, and thickness can be evaluated. The right ventricle anterior wall is located at the top of the screen and is often difficult to evaluate due to near field artifacts. The right ventricle is seen next as an echo-free space. The interventricular septum is then noted with normal motion posterior during systole and anterior during diastole.

The left ventricle is seen after the interventricular septum as another echo-free space except for an occasional linear tracing.

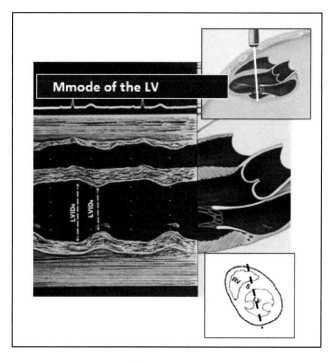

M-mode of the Left Ventricle

These linear echoes may be seen in the LV cavity or as a linear tracing adjacent to the inferolateral wall of the left ventricle and moving in the same general pattern. These are the chordae tendineae which is often mistaken for the endocardial surface of the inferolateral wall. With careful scrutiny a small echo-free space is usually seen between the chordal structures and the inferolateral wall. The normal inferolateral wall moves in an anterior direction during systole and a posterior direction during diastole. The interventricular septum and the inferolateral wall are approximately the same thickness. The pericardium is noted as an area of increased echogenicity or brightening adjacent to the normally thicker myocardium.

M-mode makes it easy to identify paradoxical motion of the septum due to elevated right heart pressures or electro physiologic dyssynchrony of the septum and inferolateral walls.

If all the wall segments are contracting equally M-mode can also be used to calculate an ejection fraction or EF% by measuring the LV Internal Diameter (ID) at end diastole and again during peak systole as illustrated in the diagram below. Although a linear measurement is being made the value is cubed to obtain a volume and is then plugged into the following formula to calculate the percentage of blood that is ejected with each beat of the heart.

FORMULA FOR CALCULATING EJECTION FRACTION:

$$EF = \frac{(LVID_{diastole})^3 - (LVID_{systole})^3}{(LVID_{diastole})^3} \times 100\%$$

The actual volume of blood that is ejected is known as stroke volume and this number multiplied times the heart rate can yield the patient's cardiac output. A Fraction Shortening can also be performed when obtaining an M-mode of the LV. The Fraction Shortening equation is just like the EF% equation but is calculating dimension instead of volume.

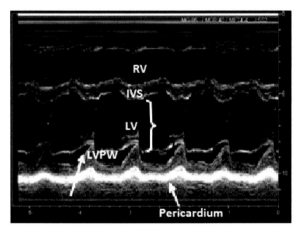

M-Mode Right and Left Ventricles

M-Mode of the Pulmonic Valve

Though rarely done anymore, M-mode tracings of the pulmonic valve may be

obtained in the parasternal short axis view. Only one leaflet is recorded. This tracing is also labeled D.E.F.A.C. as on the mitral valve. The D point is at the end of diastole or onset of systole. The E point is at the valve excursion. There is a small dip which occurs after atrial contraction or A wave and is called the A point. The C point is at the closure of the valve. When pulmonic stenosis is present the A wave is increased greater than 7 mm. When pulmonary hypertension is present the A wave is decreased less than 2 mm. Mid-systolic notching or what may be called the "Flying W" may be seen when pulmonary hypertension is present. Doppler assessment of the pulmonic valve is more commonly done

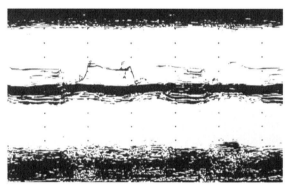

M-Mode of the Pulmonic Valve

M- Mode of the Tricuspid Valve

M-mode tracings of the tricuspid valve may also be done and look similar to that of the mitral valve, except usually only one or possibly two of the three leaflets are recorded. Similarly, because Doppler methods of evaluation of the tricuspid valve provide more quantitative information they have replaced M-mode evaluations in almost all echocardiography departments.

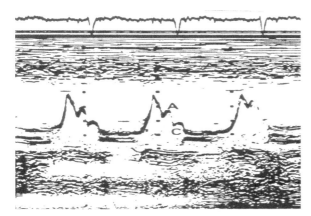

M-Mode of the Tricuspid Valve

2D Measurements

M-mode measurements have largely been replaced by 2D imaging. A parasternal long axis view is obtained and the image is frozen at end-diastole and end-systole. Measurements that are taken at end-diastole include the RV from inner-edge to inner-edge, IVS thickness, LV, LVPW thickness, aortic root measurement from either inner to inner or leading edge to leading edge. From the end-systolic frame, the LV at end-systole is measured and the left atrial from inner to inner can be measured. The volume measurement of the LA is the preferred method in determining LA size. When tracing the left atrial volume, it should be performed in the A4C and A2C chamber views when the LA is at its widest point or at end systole.

The most accurate measurement for the RV is in the A4C image.

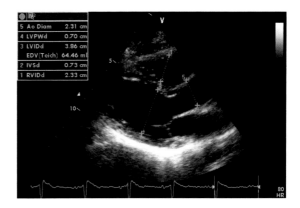

2D End-diastolic measurements

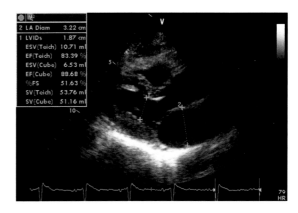

2D End-systolic measurements

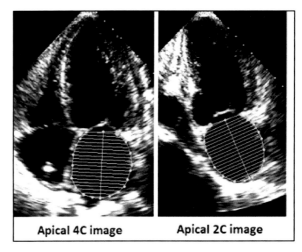

Apical 4C image   **Apical 2C image**

LA volume measurement in A4C and A2C image

53

2D Measurement	Normal Value	
RV	1.9 – 3.8 cm	
IVSd	.06 - .09 cm women	
	.06 – 1.0 cm	men
LVIDd	3.9 – 5.3 cm women	
	4.2 – 5.9 cm	men
LVPWd	.06 - .09 cm women	
	.06 – 1.0 cm	men
Aorta	1.4 – 2.6 cm annulus	
	2.1 – 3.5 cm	sinus
	2.1 – 3.4 cm ascending	
LVIDs	2.1 – 4.0 cm	
LAs	2.7 – 3.8 cm women	
	3.0 – 4.0 cm	men

2D and M-mode Normal Values

$$FS = \frac{LVIDd - LVIDS}{LVIDd} \times 100\%$$

BEST APPROACH FOR DOPPLER STUDIES

The Doppler examination of the cardiac structures has been extremely useful for the determination of valve abnormalities, congenital defects, and other flow disturbances.

Doppler of the Mitral Valve

Evaluation of the mitral valve can be achieved utilizing a variety of approaches. The apical position is usually one of the best to evaluate for mitral stenosis and mitral regurgitation because the Doppler beam is parallel to blood flow through the valve apparatus. Other windows may be useful when the jets are eccentric.

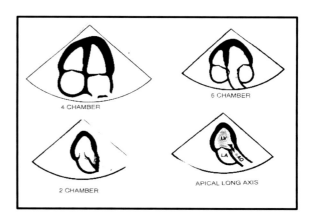

Doppler Views for Mitral Valve

With the use of conventional Doppler, as well as color flow imaging, mitral regurgitation can be evaluated by examining the flow proximal to the valve. On color flow imaging the degree of regurgitation is determined by the length, width and height of the jet. Other methods evaluate the overall jet area or a ratio of the MR jet area to the area of the left atrium. Mitral regurgitation on color flow imaging is demonstrated in shades of blue with a possible mosaic appearance that represents turbulent flow. Color gain and the color PRF settings can influence the appearance or size of the jet in color and other methods to assess MR may also be needed.

If pulsed Doppler is used, the sample gate is moved proximal to the valve and a mapping process is performed along the interatrial septum, from the valve orifice back into the left atrium, and along the left atrial wall to map the extent of the jet. Once again, the severity is based on the length, width, and height of the jet, so multiple tomographic planes are helpful. The regurgitant jet is displayed below the zero baseline on the spectral display. Continuous wave Doppler should also be used to sweep through the valve and to obtain the maximum peak velocity of the mitral regurgitant jet which typically corresponds to the center of the jet. The peak velocity does not determine the severity of MR though.

It is the density of the CW spectral display which corresponds to the number of red blood cells or volume of regurgitant flow that determines the degree of severity. Other methods of quantifying mitral regurgitation such as jet area, jet area to left atria area ratio, regurgitant fraction and PISA will be described in the section on valvular disease. Mitral regurgitation may also be detected on a parasternal long axis view, depending upon the size and position of the jet.

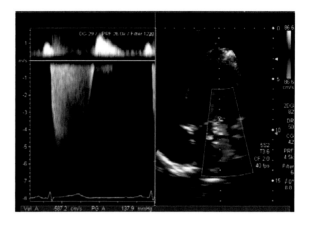

CW Doppler Mitral Regurgitation

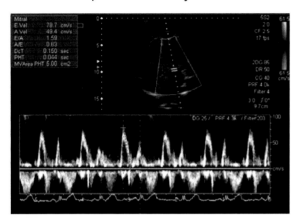

Normal Mitral Valve Flow

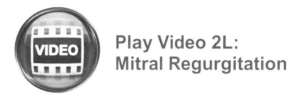

Play Video 2L:
Mitral Regurgitation

Assessment of **pulmonary vein flow** is sometimes used to determine the severity of mitral regurgitation. A combination of color flow imaging and pulsed wave Doppler can determine the location of the pulmonary veins and their flow direction in cases of severe mitral regurgitation. Reversal of pulmonary vein flow during systole is indicative of severe mitral regurgitation.

Pulmonary vein flow is also part of the criteria used to assess diastolic function. The most challenging part of assessing pulmonary vein flow is the deep imaging depth at which they are normally found behind the left atrium from an apical four chamber window. Because the pulmonary vein flow is much slower it also requires PW Doppler and lower PRF or scale settings.

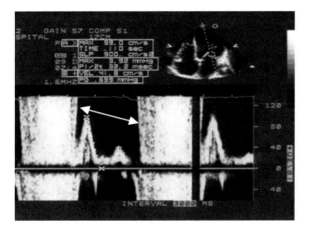

Pulsed Doppler Mitral Regurgitation

Timing of Pulmonary Vein Flow Components

- PVs₁ - early systole
- PVs₂ - mid to late systole
- PVd - during diastole after mitral valve opening
- PVa - end diastole

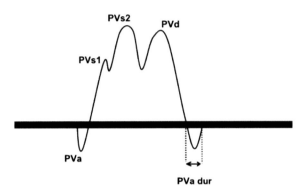

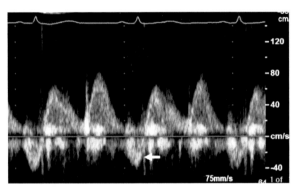

PVa duration

The PVa dur is the duration of the PVa. Since the first two parts of the signal are close together, the PVs₁ may not be seen in approximately 70% of patients with an atrioventricular conduction.

Pulmonary vein flow velocity can be obtained and analyzed in conjunction with the mitral inflow velocities for the assessment of left ventricular diastolic function.

Play Video 2M: Pulmonary Vein Flow using Color Flow and Pulmonary Vein Flow using PW Doppler

Mitral stenosis is seen on color flow imaging by the characteristic "candle-flame" appearance. This denotes the high velocity flow distal to the valve. It is necessary to use a continuous wave Doppler transducer to make sure the highest velocity flow is obtained, allowing for quantification of the stenosis and valve area. The spectral waveform will show spectral filling of the high velocity signal, and flattening of the E wave. The Doppler calculation of mitral valve area will be discussed in great detail in the section on valvular disease.

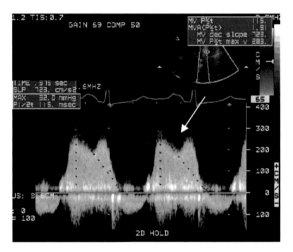

Mitral Stenosis from CW Doppler

Doppler of the Tricuspid Valve

Tricuspid regurgitation may be evaluated in the apical position similar to that of the mitral valve. Other Doppler approaches for assessing tricuspid regurgitation are the parasternal long axis inflow view, the parasternal short axis view and the subcostal view. The use of continuous wave Doppler is necessary if the tricuspid valve regurgitant jet is being obtained to calculate the right ventricular systolic pressure. Flow mapping and color techniques for the tricuspid valve are the same as the mitral valve, except it is performed on the right side of the heart.

The best approach for **tricuspid stenosis** is usually the apical, parasternal inflow, or parasternal short axis views. The peak velocity of the stenotic jet is obtained distal to the valve and calculations of valve area made.

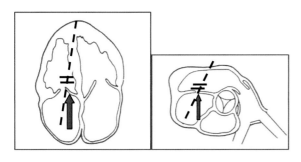

Apical 4C and PSAX view of Tricuspid Valve

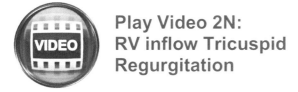

Play Video 2N: RV inflow Tricuspid Regurgitation

Doppler of the Aortic Valve

Doppler approaches to evaluate for **aortic regurgitation** are typically in the parasternal and apical positions. Color flow imaging of aortic regurgitation is displayed in red or shades of red. Color flow also helps display the jet size and direction which enables accurate placement of the CW curser to obtain the best Doppler waveform. Pulsed wave Doppler is seldom used to map Aortic Insufficiency anymore but if a PW Doppler technique is used, mapping of the jet is performed proximal to the valve in the left ventricular outflow tract, along the interventricular septum, and the anterior mitral leaflet. Once again, the severity of the jet is based on its area, height, or ratio to the left ventricular outflow tract. A spectral display of aortic regurgitation shows the jet displayed above the zero baseline. Doppler calculations may be performed to estimate

the severity of aortic regurgitation using CW Doppler and methods such as pressure half-time measurements which will be covered in the section on valvular disease.

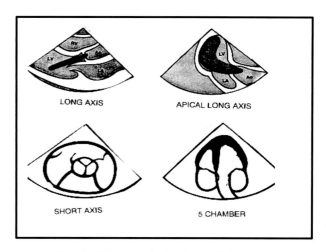

Doppler Views for Aortic Regurgitation

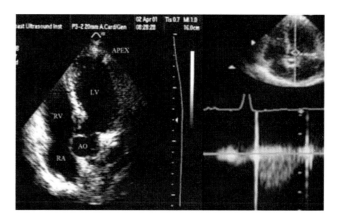

Normal Aortic Valve Flow from Apical 5C View

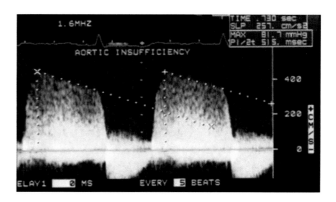

Aortic Regurgitation using CW Doppler

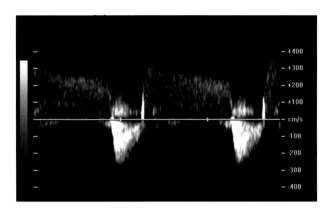

Doppler of Aortic Stenosis and Insufficiency

Aortic stenosis is evaluated best with a continuous wave Doppler. The views used are the apical, suprasternal, and right parasternal. Sometimes the subcostal view may be helpful. The peak velocity of the stenotic jet needs to be obtained distal to the valve. Aortic valve area and peak and mean pressure gradients can be obtained. The ASE recommends utilizing a "blind,non-imaging" PEDOF CW transducer to ensure obtaining the highest velocity from the stenotic jet.

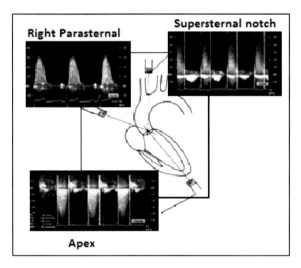

Doppler Views for Aortic Stenosis using Pedof probe

Due to potential jet eccentricity (see diagram below) all the various sites should be interrogated to acquire the highest velocity waveform.

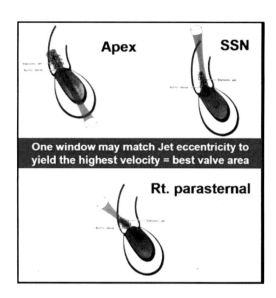

PEDOF CW probe windows for Aortic Stenosis

Failure to obtain the highest actual velocity could result in underestimation of the severity of stenosis by over estimating the aortic valve area.

Doppler of the Pulmonic Valve

The Doppler approach to evaluate for **pulmonic regurgitation** is the parasternal short axis at the AV level or parasternal long axis of the right ventricular outflow view. If a right ventricular systolic pressure measurement is being performed, continuous wave Doppler should be used. Otherwise color flow imaging and pulsed or CW Doppler can be utilized to evaluate pulmonic regurgitation. Color flow imaging displays pulmonic regurgitation in red or shades of red as represented by flow towards the transducer. Pulmonic regurgitation is seen in the right ventricular outflow tract and can be mapped with pulsed Doppler along the anterior aortic root wall, through the middle of the outflow tract, and along the anterior outflow tract wall.

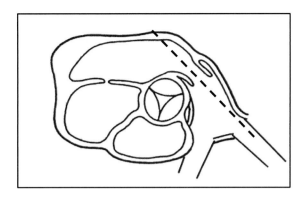

Doppler View for Pulmonic Valve - PSAX

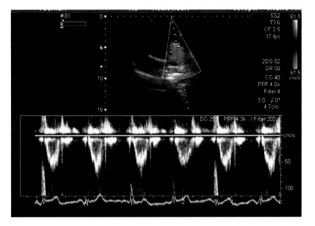

Normal Pulmonic Valve Flow using PW

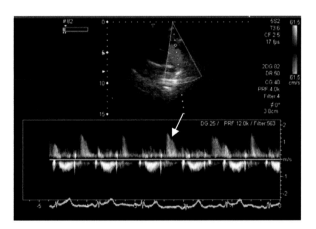

Pulmonic Valve Regurgitation using CW

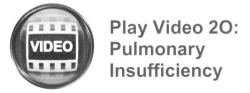

Play Video 2O:
Pulmonary
Insufficiency

Pulmonic stenosis is also best assessed in this view. The highest velocity jet will be found distal to the valve unless infundibular stenosis is suspected. The pulmonic valve may sometimes be evaluated in the subcostal view.

Other Doppler Uses

Multiple Doppler sites may be used for evaluating **ventricular septal defects**. The parasternal long and short axis, or subcostal views are often the most helpful. The parasternal views are often best when using continuous wave Doppler to obtain the peak velocity of the shunt since those views provide the angle to flow closest to zero. The best views to determine **atrial septal defects** are the parasternal short axis, apical and subcostal views. The subcostal view is typically the best view to evaluate the interatrial septum, but it cannot always be obtained on every patient. The Doppler views to evaluate a patient for a **patent ductus arteriosus** are the parasternal short axis view and suprasternal view.

Subaortic stenosis from asymmetrical septal hypertrophy may be detected in the parasternal views or apical views. The apical five chamber, or apical long axis views are typically best for pulsed wave Doppler mapping from the apex through the LVOT to determine the actual site of obstruction. CW is then activated to quantify the pressure gradient from the obstruction. M-mode is used from the parasternal long-axis view to determine if there is SAM, Systolic Anterior Motion of the mitral leaflet which contributes to obstructing the LVOT, a premature closure of the AV, and a very abrupt end to systole creating a stroke volume with a smaller or very small amount of blood being ejected.

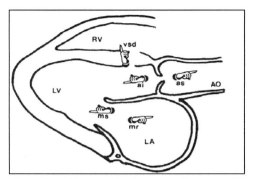

Parasternal Long-axis view - membranous VSD & flow abnormalities.

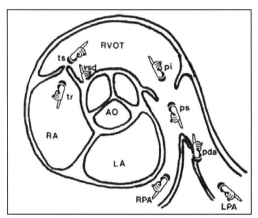

Parasternal Short-axis view at AV level - membranous VSD & flow abnormalities.

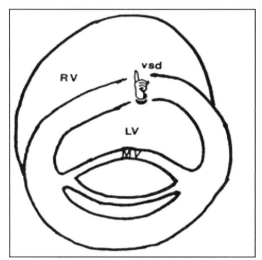

Parasternal Short-axis view at LV level - muscular VSD

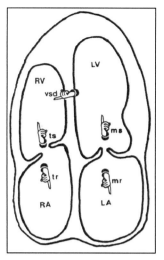

Apical 4C view with shunts and flow abnormalities.

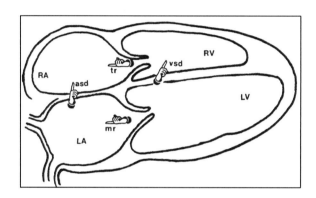

Subcostal view with shunts & flow abnormalities

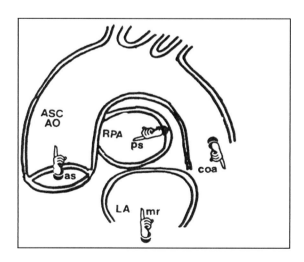

Suprasternal notch view of shunts and flow abnormalities.

DOPPLER OVERVIEW

Doppler is another function used in echocardiography. Johan Christian Doppler is responsible for the theory of the Doppler effect. When applied to the heart, the Doppler effect is enacted when ultrasound waves which are sent from the transducer to the heart are reflected back to the transducer by the moving red blood cells in the heart. The difference between the transmitted frequency and the reflected frequency is the Doppler shift. In echocardiography this Doppler shift is in the audible range of sound and can be heard by the operator and the information received by the transducer can determine the speed and direction of flow.

There are two types of Doppler used in echocardiography. Pulsed Wave (PW) and Continuous Wave (CW) Doppler. Pulsed wave Doppler utilizes one piezoelectric element that sends and receives sound. Because both functions are shared by one element, a pulsed Doppler transducer has a pulse repetition frequency. The pulse repetition frequency is the frequency at which the transducer switches from sending to receiving sound.

There are advantages and disadvantages to pulsed Doppler. The advantages are the use of a sample gate or sample volume which is defined along the Doppler cursor providing range resolution. This allows site specific flow information to be obtained. Pulsed Doppler can also be used simultaneously with real time imaging. The disadvantages result from the pulse repetition frequency. Pulsed Doppler transducers have a Nyquist limit. The Nyquist limit is reached when the Doppler shift equals or exceeds one-half of the pulse repetition frequency. If the pulse repetition frequency is exceeded, the Doppler signal will alias. Aliasing is an artifact caused by a wrapping around of the Doppler signal. For this reason, continuous wave Doppler is also used.

Continuous wave Doppler uses two separate crystals or elements. One that sends sound and one that receives sound. This eliminates aliasing since there is no pulse repetition frequency, however, there is range ambiguity. Continuous wave Doppler has been integrated with 2-dimensional echo, but does not allow for simultaneous, *live* real time and Doppler. When the Doppler mode is active the B-mode image is frozen. The 2D image may be updated automatically at preset intervals or manually by selecting a B pause or update control that switches which modality is active.

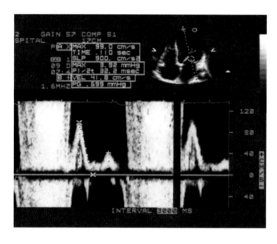

Aliasing of Mitral Regurgitation with Pulsed Doppler

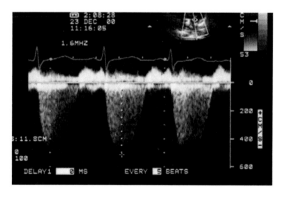

Aliasing Corrected with Continuous Wave Doppler

Color flow imaging is a form of pulsed Doppler. Information is obtained from multiple sample gates. The colors are assigned to the frequency shifts of the sound waves reflected from the red blood cells. Since color flow imaging is achieved by a series of Doppler pulses, when ultrasound is sent into the tissue along a given line, it is reflected back to the transducer at incremented times. This method allows for receiving information all along the line, whereas conventional pulsed Doppler ignores everything along the line except for where the range or sample gate is placed.

In color flow imaging the machine collects amplitude and phase shifted information at all the sample sites. A quadrature detector determines flow direction information and autocorrelation is used to analyze velocity information. The auto correlator does a comparison of the returning signal frequency to the transmitted signal frequency and assigns a color value to the differences. Color is assigned based on three principles: blood flow direction, mean velocity of the blood flow, and the variance of detected frequency shifts or non-laminar flow.

The colors red, blue, and green are traditionally used in color flow imaging. Several map and color variations have been incorporated into systems. The acronym **BART** is used for the color display for cardiac applications meaning ***Blue Away Red Towards*** the transducer. In other words, flow towards the transducer is displayed in varying shades of red based on the returning Doppler shift. As flow velocities increase the shades get lighter. Flow away from the transducer is displayed in shades of blue. As velocities get higher the shades get lighter.

Although the color display can be inverted this function is not used for cardiac applications making color detection of regurgitant jets much easier. Many maps have colors such as yellow incorporated within them. The color green is used to show non-laminar flow or turbulence. This may be referred to as variance. Variance is the deviation between

two frequency shifts of two consecutive transmitted bursts along a given scan line. A mosaic pattern is noted on color flow imaging as a result of the wide range of velocities and non-laminar flow. A mosaic or confetti appearance is a combination of shades of white, green, red, yellow and blue-cyan.

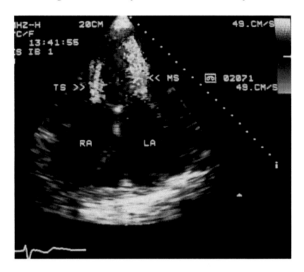

CFI of Mitral and Tricuspid Stenosis

Advantages of color flow imaging are accuracy of detecting high velocity jets and regurgitant lesions. As discussed earlier it also shows flow characteristics such as turbulence and also timing and duration of events according to the cardiac cycle. It makes the exam more efficient since detection of the disease is easier and it allows for a spatial display.

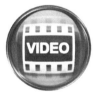

Play Video 2P: CFI Apical Long Axis of AI Jet showing it distinctly from Mitral Inflow.

Disadvantages are those similar to conventional pulsed wave Doppler. It should be mentioned though that Pulsed and CW Doppler spectral waveforms have better temporal resolution with regard to timing and duration of events.

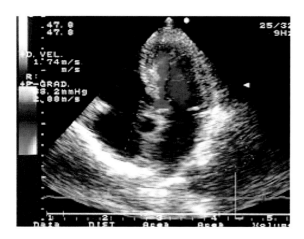

Color uses an overlay technique which can include segments of both systole and diastole.

Color only shows a mean velocity so it is much less quantitative than spectral Doppler for measuring pressure gradients and the severity of certain lesions or for determining valve area. This also means that color will alias sooner or at lower velocities than conventional pulsed Doppler techniques and therefore aliasing does not indicate by itself that pathology is present. Other methods need to be employed to confirm or rule out disease or to assess severity.

TRANSESOPHAGEAL ECHOCARDIOGRAPHY

Transesophageal echocardiography is performed by inserting a transducer through an endoscope into the patient's esophagus. Transesophageal echo can obtain high resolution images of the cardiac structures. The transducer is located close to the heart and utilizes higher frequency transducers than conventional transthoracic imaging. There are several types of transesophageal transducers available. Some have fixed imaging planes such as bi-plane transducers while the newer ones are omniplane or multiplane allowing for more image acquisition and some also include 3D capabilities. The transesophageal echocardiogram is still limited by factors such as patient condition, cardiac anatomy, and technical problems inherent to the technology.

Transesophageal echocardiography is used for a variety of reasons. The following table lists the more common indications for transesophageal echocardiography.

Common Indications for Transesophageal Echocardiography
• Source of embolism
• Valvular Disease
• Prosthetic Valve Function/Dysfunction
• Evaluation of aortic(aneurysm/dissection)
• Congenital heart disease
• Operative procedures or monitoring
• Intracardiac Mass
• Endocarditis (suspected)
• Other

The transesophageal probe is manipulated by rotating, angulating or tilting in order to obtain multiple images of the anatomy of the heart. The four windows that are obtained in TEE imaging are: upper esophageal, mid esophageal, transgastric and deep transgastric planes. It is imperative that the sonographer know all the anatomy when assisting with the TEE.

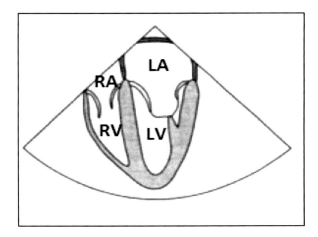

Mid Esophageal Apical 4C view with TEE

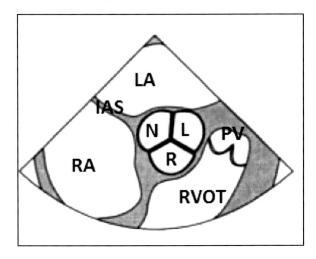

Mid Esophageal Aortic Valve Short Axis View

When performing a TEE, the order should be verified before beginning the study. The patient should by NPO for at least 4 – 6 hours prior to the examination. A patient history should be taken to verify any difficulty shallowing, allergies, history of bleeding disorder or any other medical conditions. The procedure should be explained and a consent form must be signed. All dentures must be removed from the patient. If the patient has permanent teeth, a bite block is placed to help protect the probe and the patient. The patient is given IV sedation and rolled into the left lateral position. Post procedure, the patient should be monitored for at least 30 minutes to verify all vital signs are within normal limits and there is no evidence of esophageal bleeding.

The TEE probe should be examined for any cracks or tears, rinsed with soap and then soaked in a disinfecting solution for at least 20 minutes. After the probe has been soaked, it should be rinsed and stored in an appropriate hanging rack to assure the probe does not get kinked or bent. Bending the probe may cause damage.

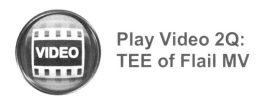

Play Video 2Q: TEE of Flail MV

USE OF CONTRAST AGENTS

Contrast agents have been used for over thirty years in conjunction with echocardiography. Some newer agents have been approved and others are pending approval for use in echocardiography. The FDA rquires contrast agents carry a "black box warning" that advises the potential risk of serious cardiac injuries and death. This has affected its widespread utilization to enhance imaging in echocardiography examinations that would otherwise be equivocal or non-diagnostic and require other costly modalities to render a diagnosis. Many examiners have petitioned the FDA to remove the "black box warning" stating "withholding these agents would make diagnosis of life- threatening heart disease more difficult." Recent articles have outlined a protocol for allowing use of contrast on selected patients.

Contrast agents help to identify specific cardiac anomalies and improve image quality. Saline has been one of the most commonly used contrast agents in echocardiography until recently. Agitated saline is injected into the venous system while cardiac imaging is performed. The air- filled microbubbles are very reflective and are easily detected entering the right side of the heart. This technique has primarily been used to help detect and assess cardiac shunts or evaluate right heart structures. The biggest limitation to saline only contrast is the short duration of the microbubbles.

Play Video 2R: Contrast study for ASD

The newer contrast agents produce microbubbles that either have low solubility gases, or surface stabilizing shells, or both. These contrast agents coupled with harmonic imaging allows for better visualization of the contrast and longer lasting bubbles. These agents help to identify the border between the myocardium and blood flow by opacifying the left ventricle cavity, allowing assessment of global and regional systolic function of the left ventricle. Additional uses of contrast agents include: help for the identification of altered cardiovascular anatomy, complications of myocardial infarction, and enhanced detection of a suspected ascending aortic aneurysm during transesophageal echocardiography.

Contrast agents have significantly improved the diagnostic capabilities of stress echocardiography and helps to enhance Doppler signals that may otherwise go un-detected.

Future applications of contrast agents include myocardial perfusion detection, assessment of the coronary vasculature, endothelial function, and therapeutic uses.

Spontaneous contrast is found in patients with slow moving blood flow with very low cardiac output. The visualization of the red blood cells on the conventional echocardiogram is the result of the clumping of the cells together allowing for reflection of the ultrasound beam. The sonographer should always look for the presence of a clot if spontaneous contrast is seen.

PROVOCATIVE MANEUVERS

Provocative maneuvers are used in echocardiography to determine certain conditions in the heart or enhance them. The Valsalva maneuver which is performed by having the patient exhale and "holding" it out which causes an increase in the intra-thoracic pressure and decreases pre-loading conditions by decreasing venous return. This maneuver slows the pulse down and by decreasing blood returning to the heart it creates an increase in venous pressure. This may cause an augmentation of mitral valve prolapse or provoke one. This maneuver may also cause an increase in the obstruction in patients with a hypertrophic cardiomyopathy.

Amyl nitrate is a vasodilator and may be given to patients to provoke or augment mitral valve prolapse or obstruction due to hypertrophic cardiomyopathy.

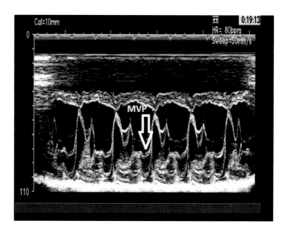

Mitral Valve Prolapse

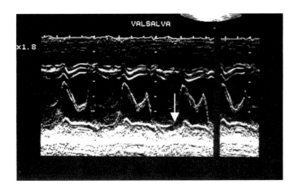

Prolapse Augmented with Valsalva

Isometric handgrips can be used to cause an acute increase in blood pressure. The use of these handgrips may help to augment jets of mitral and aortic regurgitation. Isometric handgrips may also be used to detect or produce wall motion abnormalities.

Straight leg raises performed by the patient may augment tricuspid regurgitation by increasing venous return. Other forms of stressing cardiac patients will be discussed in a dedicated portion of this workbook on Stress Testing.

CPR

Cardiopulmonary resuscitation is the administering of emergency medical care to someone who is unconscious. The cardiac and pulmonary functions should be assessed quickly to see if CPR is necessary. The goal of CPR is to provide oxygen to the brain, heart, and other vital organs until medical treatment is available. If spinal or head trauma is suspected, do not move the person unless absolutely necessary.

If a person is found unconscious, the first step is to establish if the patient is responsive. If an adult patient is found to be unresponsive, emergency medical services should be alerted and then CPR begun. If no spinal or head injury is present or suspected, the patient is placed in a supine position and the head should be tilted back, helping to open the airway. The mouth and throat should be checked for any liquid or solid material and cleared if possible. Listen and look for signs of breathing. Watch for the rise and fall of the chest. If the patient is breathless, rescue breathing is begun.

Pinch the victims nose. The rescuer takes a large breath in and places their mouth completely over the victim's mouth creating an airtight seal. Two full breaths are given, each taking 1 to 1 1/2 seconds. Make sure the victim's chest rises indicating proper ventilation. Too much air may cause air to go into the stomach instead of the lungs. If ventilation does not occur, the Heimlich maneuver may be necessary to clear the airway of foreign bodies. If possible, a bag-valve-mask or other type device should be used to prevent transmission of disease.

Circulation can be assessed by checking the carotid artery pulse. The carotid artery is located between the trachea and strap muscles in the neck. If a pulse cannot be located, assume the victim is in cardiac arrest. Chest compressions and breathing maneuvers should be implemented. Two initial breaths are given. The rhythmic compression with the heels of the hand in the lower sternum are done.

The rescuers elbows are locked and arms extended straight. Each thrust should be straight down on the victim's chest. The chest should be compressed 1 ½" to 2" for an adult and 1" to 1 ½" on a child. An infant's chest should be compressed no more than ½" to 1" inch by using two fingers rather than the palm of the hand. The chest should return to normal after each compression. This allows flow back into the heart.

Compression rates are 80 to 100 per minute for an adult and at least 100 per minute for a child. If one person is performing the CPR, 30 compressions are performed for every 2 breaths. The same procedure is applied when there are two rescuers performing CPR. This is done until advanced cardiac life support can be administered.

TECHNIQUE QUIZ

1. The gain control provides what function?
   a. rectification of sound pulse
   b. incremental power adjustment
   c. amplification of returning signal
   d. reduced sound beam divergence

2. The intensity of the sound beam is controlled by:
   a. overall gain
   b. transmit power
   c. changing transducer frequency
   d. pulse repetition frequency

3. The resonant frequency of a transducer is its:
   a. peak frequency
   b. operating frequency
   c. propagation frequency
   d. lowest frequency

4. What is the greatest advantage of utilizing pulsed wave Doppler?
   a. lack of aliasing
   b. sensitivity to high velocity flow
   c. range resolution
   d. uses two crystals instead of one

5. Which of the following is not a limitation of continuous wave Doppler?
   a. aliasing
   b. simultaneous Doppler and B-mode
   c. range resolution
   d. Inherent Spectral broadening

6. The Nyquist limit is equal to _____ the pulse repetition frequency.
   a. 1/4
   b. 1/3
   c. 1/2
   d. 2 times

7. Which statement about color flow imaging is most correct?
   a. CFI provides as much quantitative information as PW spectral analysis
   b. CFI provides spatial flow information and mean velocity than PW spectral analysis
   c. Color flow is processed by a FFT technique
   d. None of the above are correct

8. What does the quadrature detector determines in color flow imaging?
   a. frequency of sound
   b. amplification of sound
   c. flow direction
   d. Nyquist limit

9. The color green in the color flow display depicts:
   a. laminar flow
   b. non-laminar flow
   c. plug flow
   d. low flow

10. Frame rate can be increased the MOST by:
    a. decreasing the sector depth
    b. decreasing the sector width
    c. eliminating one focal zone
    d. increasing the pulse repetition frequency

11. Which of the following will NOT help to correct aliasing?
    a. increasing the pulse repetition frequency
    b. adjust the zero baseline
    c. use continuous wave Doppler
    d. increasing transducer frequency

12. The apical long axis view is used because:
    a. it visualizes the antero-septal and inferior-lateral walls of the left ventricle
    b. it is parallel to flow for the MV, LVOT and aortic valve
    c. it visualizes structures not seen from any other window
    d. it provides the best view of the right ventricle and intraventricular septum

13. The smallest to largest group of intensities that produce a shade of gray on the monitor describes the:
    a. dynamic range
    b. range equation
    c. Nyquist limit
    d. temporal resolution

14. An acoustic shadow is caused when the ultrasound beam encounters:
    a. low attenuating fluid
    b. dense objects that attenuate sound
    c. a medium with a different speed of sound
    d. specular reflectors

15. A mitral valve prolapse may be augmented by having the patient:
    a. inspire
    b. lie very flat
    c. perform a Valsalva maneuver
    d. placed in Trendelenburg position

16. Inhaling amyl nitrite may help to provoke or enhance:
    a. mitral valve prolapse
    b. the obstruction in patients with a sub-aortic stenosis
    c. neither condition
    d. both conditions

17. Spontaneous contrast is due to all of the following except:
    a. Low cardiac output
    b. Slow moving red blood cells
    c. Increased reflection from clumps of red blood cells
    d. Shunting from high pressure to low pressure chamber

18. What type of cardiac flow abnormality is displayed on the Doppler/image below:
    a. aortic regurgitation
    b. mitral regurgitation
    c. tricuspid regurgitation
    d. pulmonic regurgitation

19. The brief appearance of large patterns of B&W or color displayed over anatomic structures that are not related to any associated flow patterns describes what type of artifact?
    a. ghosting
    b. side lobe
    c. aliasing
    d. color speckle or noise

20. M-mode samples at a rate of:
    a. 1200 frames per second
    b. 30 frames per second
    c. 1800 frames per second
    d. 18 frames per second

21. The A wave on the M-mode tracing of the mitral valve represents:
    a. maximum anterior leaflet excursion
    b. atrial contraction
    c. end diastole
    d. when to measure for largest left atrial dimension

22. A "B" bump or notch on the mitral valve M-mode tracing may indicate:
    a. mitral stenosis
    b. systolic anterior motion
    c. mitral regurgitation
    d. elevated left ventricular end diastolic pressure

23. Which of the following is NOT a direct cause for an increased EPSS?
    a. dilated left ventricle
    b. aortic stenosis
    c. mitral stenosis
    d. aortic regurgitation

24. What structure on the M-mode tracing of the left ventricle is often mistaken for the endocardial surface?
    a. posterior mitral valve leaflet
    b. anterior mitral valve leaflet
    c. chordae tendineae
    d. pericardium

25. Premature closure of the AV on the M-mode tracing may represent:
    a. systemic hypertension
    b. pulmonic hypertension
    c. increased cardiac output
    d. sub-valvular (AV) obstruction

26. If a "flying W" or mid-systolic notching is seen on the pulmonic valve M-mode tracing, it may indicate:
    a. portal hypertension
    b. pulmonary hypertension
    c. pulmonic stenosis
    d. pulmonic regurgitation

27. Which statement about Doppler evaluation of pulmonary veins is MOST correct?
    a. Deep imaging depth requires use of CW or aliasing occurs
    b. Best visualized from the apical 2 chamber view
    c. Systolic flow reversal is indicative of severe mitral regurgitation
    d. Requires limited adjustment of PRF

28. Name the anatomy labeled by the "X" in the TEE image:

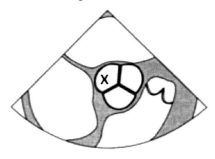

    a. RCC of the aorta
    b. Anterior mitral valve
    c. NCC of the aorta
    d. LCC of the pulmonic valve

29. The proper compression to ventilation ratio for two rescuer CPR on an adult victim is:
    a. 30-2
    b. 5-2
    c. 5-1
    d. 15-1

30. What structure is indicated by the arrow on the M-mode tracing below:
    a. interventricular septum
    b. inferolateral/ posterior wall
    c. chordae tendineae
    d. endocardium

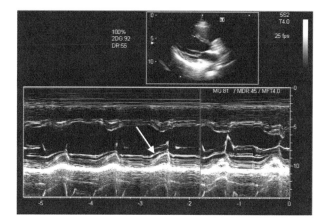

31. What artifact is displayed on the spectral analysis image below?
    a. mirror imaging
    b. aliasing
    c. range ambiguity
    d. reverberation

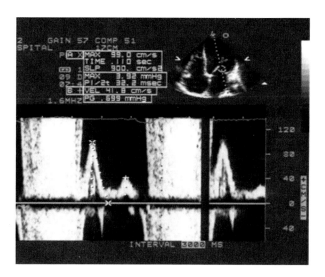

32. What type of filter permits the frequencies to be transmitted that are above where the filter is tuned?
    a. low pass
    b. pass band
    c. high pass
    d. stop band

33. What view is demonstrated in the image below?
    a. subcostal
    b. suprasternal
    c. parasternal short axis
    d. apical long axis

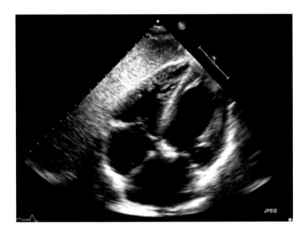

34. How would you obtain an A2C view from an A4C view?
    a. aim more anteriorly in the chest
    b. rotate the transducer degrees clockwise
    c. rotate the transducer 45 degrees counter clockwise
    d. aim more posteriorly in the chest

35. What wall of the heart is indicated by the arrow on the apical 2 chamber image below?
    a. anterior wall
    b. inferior wall
    c. interventricular septal wall
    d. lateral wall

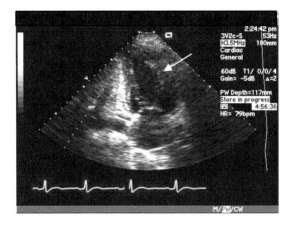

36. What coronary feeds the heart wall indicated by the arrow in the following echo image?
    a. Diagonal
    b. RCA
    c. Left Circumflex
    d. Left Anterior Descending

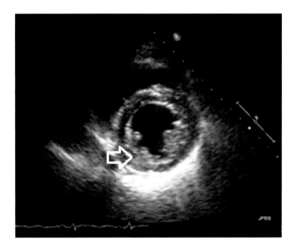

37. What anatomy is indicated by the arrow in the following echo image?

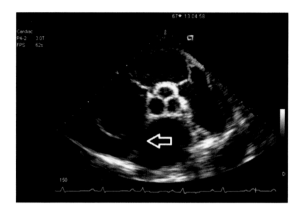

   a. LA appendage
   b. IAS
   c. IVS
   d. RVOT

38. What piece of equipment is used to protect the TEE probe and the patient when the patient has teeth?

   a. Nasal cannula
   b. Bite block
   c. Suction
   d. Tongue blade

39. What function can be performed to avoid aliasing in the following Doppler image?

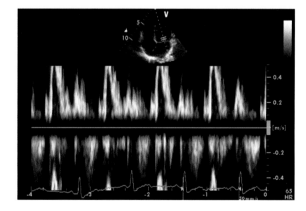

   a. increase velocity scale
   b. decrease velocity scale
   c. shift baseline up
   d. decrease overall gain

40. Identify the numbered locations with the following options:

   __ Left Ventricle
   __ Left Atrium
   __ Antero-septal wall
   __ Right Coronary Cusp

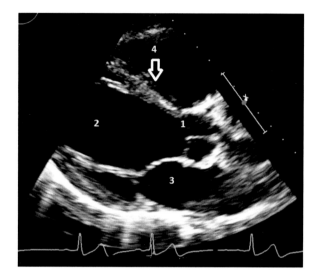

41. What occurs during the holding phase of Valsalva maneuver?
   a. Increase venous return
   b. Increase aortic pressure
   c. Decrease venous return
   d. Decrease aortic pressure

42. The TEE probe should be stored:

   a. In a sterile environment
   b. Coiled in a box
   c. In an appropriate rack with the probe hanging down
   d. It doesn't matter

43. Name the image shown in the scan below?
    a. Apical 4C
    b. Parasternal short axis aortic level
    c. Parasternal long axis
    d. Right ventricular inflow tract

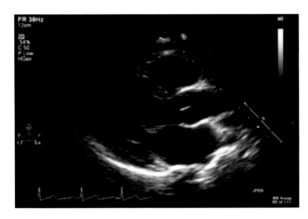

44. Identify at what location you would perform a peak velocity measurement of the mitral valve:

    a. 1
    b. 2
    c. 3
    d. 4

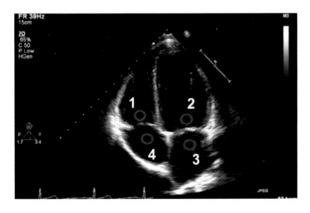

45. A LVPW/Inferolateral wall thickness measurement of 15 mm indicates:
    a. Normal wall thickness
    b. LVH
    c. RVH
    d. Abnormal wall thinning

46. A LVIDd value of 6.2 cm is considered:
    a. Normal
    b. Small
    c. Dilated
    d. None of the above

47. What is the FS% for the given information:
    LVIDd   55 mm
    LVIDs   32 mm

    a. .42
    b. 23
    c. .34
    d. 42

48. Diagnose the following M-mode:
    a. Hyperdynamic LV
    b. Reduced cardiac output
    c. Aortic stenosis
    d. Pericardial effusion

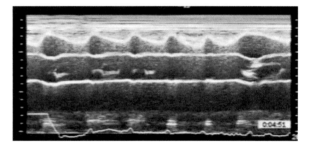

49. When performing a TEE, the patient should be in this position?
    a. right lateral
    b. supine
    c. left lateral
    d. prone

50. What two views can you visualize the left atrial appendage?
    a. PLA and PSA at aortic level
    b. A4C and A2C
    c. PSA at the aortic level and A2C
    d. A2C and A3C

51. Name the anatomy marked by the "X":
    a. Right common carotid
    b. Brachiocephalic
    c. Left Common Carotid
    d. Left Subclavian

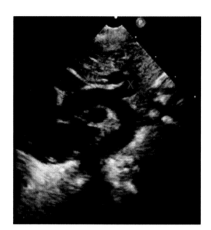

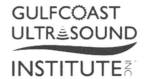

Section 3:

Valvular Heart Disease

Section 3: VALVULAR HEART DISEASE

Objectives

Upon completion of this module you should be able to:

- Identify normal anatomy of the cardiac valves
- Recognize abnormal findings associated with valvular disease on the two-dimensional, M-mode, and Doppler examination
- Outline physiology and hemodynamics of the cardiac valves affected by various diseases
- Recognize various commonly seen valvular diseases
- Apply various cardiac imaging and Doppler techniques
- Implement the various measuring techniques used to assess valvular heart disease
- State etiologies and clinical symptoms of the various valvular anomalies
- Recognize the affects various valvular diseases have on specific cardiac chambers and vessels
- Apply the proper techniques for the identification of endocarditis
- Recognize the various types of prosthetic heart valves
- Apply proper imaging and Doppler techniques used to evaluate prosthetic heart valves

VALVULAR HEART DISEASE

MITRAL VALVE
Physiology & Hemodynamics

The mitral valve is an atrioventricular valve that regulates blood flow from the left atria into the left ventricle. The normal mitral valve opens during diastole and closes during systole in response to changes in pressure between the left atrium and left ventricle.

At end systole, when ventricular contraction is complete, the pressure in the left ventricle drops to approximately 0-5 mmHg. Because the pressure in the left atria is higher at 10-12 mmHg since it has been filling during systole, the increased pressure in the atria forces the MV open and the *passive* or *early filling* phase of diastole begins for the left ventricle.

When the pressure begins to equalize between the two chambers the mitral valve begins to close (but not completely) and this phase of diastole is called diastasis. This phase continues until atrial contraction or atrial systole occurs which is responsible for the last 20-30% of ventricular filling.

After atrial contraction the ventricular pressure is considerably higher than the atrial pressure so the mitral valve now closes completely and should remain closed throughout systole. There are three phases to diastole: 1) Rapid filling, 2) Slow filling (diastasis) and, 3) Atrial systole. These phases of diastole are what create the M shape to the atrioventricular valves.

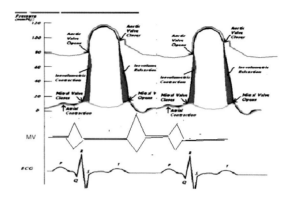

Diagram of pressure changes & phases of diastole

There is a short interval of diastole called **isovolumetric relaxation time (IVRT)** between the end of systole and the closure of the aortic valve, and just before the onset of ventricular filling and the opening of the mitral valve. Similarly, there is a brief period or phase between the closure of the mitral valve and before the opening of the aortic valve which is referred to as **isovolumetric contraction time (IVCT).**

The flow across the mitral valve during diastole corresponds to left ventricle inflow and has two corresponding peaks. The *E wave* reflects passive or early filling velocity and the *A wave* reflects the late filling velocity from atrial contraction. More details about left ventricle inflow and diastolic function of the left ventricle will be discussed in the Doppler evaluation of the Mitral Valve.

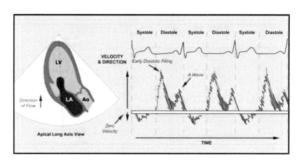

Left Ventricle Inflow through Mitral Valve

79

The mitral valve is composed of mitral leaflet tissue, papillary muscles, chordae tendineae, left ventricle myocardium, and the fibromuscular mitral annulus. In order for the mitral valve to retain its integrity, all of these components must work properly and together.

The mitral valve has two leaflets, the anterior and posterior leaflets. The mitral valve funnels blood to the aorta, permits flow from the left atrium to the left ventricle during diastole, and prevents systolic regurgitation into the left atrium. The anterior leaflet is somewhat long and triangular in shape while the posterior leaflet is shorter, but is attached to the mitral annulus more extensively. Both leaflets have a roughened surface distally where they insert with the chordae tendineae.

Arising from the anterolateral and inferomedial papillary muscles, the chordae tendineae insert into the mitral leaflets at the roughened area and free edge of the leaflets. The chordae that arise from the anterolateral papillary muscle anchors the lateral half of both leaflets and the chordae arising from the inferomedial papillary muscle anchors the medial half of the anterior and posterior mitral leaflets. Hence, the leaflets share both papillary muscles.

Mitral stenosis is the narrowing of the mitral valve orifice. There are several etiologies that can result in mitral stenosis, however, the most common cause in the adult population is rheumatic fever. Signs and symptoms of Mitral stenosis include: dyspnea on exertion (80%), hemoptysis, chest pain, palpitations, syncope, heart failure and right heart failure. During auscultation an opening snap may be heard at the apex. Rheumatic fever results in inflammation of the leaflets, commissures, and chordae tendineae, causing thickening and fibrosis. The chordal structures become shortened

and over time the fibrotic areas may develop calcific deposits.

The fibrosis and matting of the chordae tendineae create a funnel effect that also increases the stenosis. Enhancing the process further are the involvement of the papillary muscles and the mitral valve annulus Advanced cases of mitral stenosis involve the whole mitral valve apparatus resulting in little movement to allow blood to pass from the left atrium to the left ventricle during diastole. A frequent comorbidity of mitral stenosis is mitral regurgitation.

Limiting flow from the left atrium to the left ventricle results in elevated diastolic left atrial pressure greater than the left ventricle end diastolic pressure. Normally in diastole there is slightly higher left atrial to left ventricular pressure, allowing normal blood flow from the left atrium to the left ventricle followed by the equalization of pressures at end-diastole.

When mitral stenosis is present, the pressure in the left atrium stays elevated through most of diastole. The pressure difference from the left atrium to the left ventricle end diastolic pressure is called the pressure gradient. The higher the gradient, the more severe the stenosis. This also means the more severe the mitral stenosis, the higher the left atrial pressure. As a result, the pulmonary veins and capillary pressures become elevated eventually resulting in pulmonary edema and congestive heart failure. Pulmonary hypertension is another possible sequelae of mitral stenosis. Pulmonary hypertension is a result of pulmonary arteriole constriction, and is sometimes referred to as the second obstruction of mitral stenosis. Pulmonary artery pressures are often equal to or greater than systemic values in patients with chronic mitral stenosis. Pulmonary hypertension also results in dilatation of the right ventricle, right ventricular hypertrophy, tricuspid regurgitation, and elevated right atrial pressures and central venous pressure.

Other sequelae of mitral stenosis include:
1) Low cardiac output is one result of mitral stenosis. Exercise augments the hemodynamic event.
2) Enlargement of the left atrium often causes atrial fibrillation.
3) Enlargement of the left atrium and inadequate movement of blood from the left atrium results in stasis of blood.

These factors coupled with atrial fibrillation, increase the risk for a thromboembolic event.

Etiologies of mitral stenosis other than rheumatic valve disease are mitral annular calcification, congenital mitral stenosis, and obstruction of the mitral valve orifice by a mass.

Congenital mitral stenosis is uncommon. There are two major forms of congenital mitral stenosis; mitral arcade and parachute mitral valve. Mitral arcade occurs when the leaflets are fused at the commissures. The chordae are short or nonexistent. This type is similar to rheumatic mitral stenosis hemodynamically and anatomically.

The parachute deformity of the mitral valve is the other more common type of mitral valve stenosis. This occurs when there is only one papillary muscle in the left ventricle. Both chordae insert into one muscle. Obligatory blood flow is between the interchordal spaces. Narrowing of these spaces results in mitral stenosis. There are three other obstructive processes that commonly occur with a parachute mitral valve, they are: supravalvular ring of the left atrium, subaortic stenosis, and coarctation of the aorta.

Other less common types of congenital mitral stenosis usually involve shortened

chordae and papillary muscle hypertrophy and mitral hypoplasia/atresia.

Mitral annular calcifications are calcific deposits which occur on the fibrosa of the mitral ring. In mild forms they usually appear at the base of the posterior leaflet on the left ventricular side. As the disease progresses a semicircle area of increased echogenicity is seen on the posterior annulus. When calcifications become large enough or begin to involve the mitral valve leaflets, mitral stenosis can occur. Approximately 50% of patients with mitral annular calcifications have associated mitral regurgitation. More common to females, mitral annular calcifications are typically considered a degenerative, age related condition. Other conditions that may result in mitral annular calcification are metabolic diseases such as diabetes and azotemia, certain cardiomyopathies as well as increased mechanical stress on the mitral valve resulting from mitral valve prolapse or hypertension. Possible side effects are atrial arrhythmias and thromboembolic disease. Thromboembolism may arise from the left atrium or the embolization of calcium deposits.

Mitral valve orifice **obstruction** may also occur due to obstruction by a mass or tumor, most commonly an atrial myxoma. Atrial myxomas are tumors that are often connected by a stalk to the interatrial septum and may move from the left atrium into the mitral valve orifice causing obstruction of flow.

M-Mode

The echocardiographic features of mitral stenosis are often very specific on the M-mode exam. One of the most common early signs is flattening of the E-F slope. This is a result of the persistent left atrial to left ventricular pressure gradient during diastole.

Another M-mode finding is the movement of the posterior leaflet in the same direction as the anterior leaflet in diastole caused by adhesions between the edges of the leaflets. The mitral leaflets themselves will also appear thickened. The D-E distance is reduced as a result of decreased leaflet excursion. If pulmonary hypertension is present, the pulmonic valve may be thick. The A wave excursion will be reduced and mid systolic notching or a "Flying W" may be seen on the m-mode of the pulmonic valve.

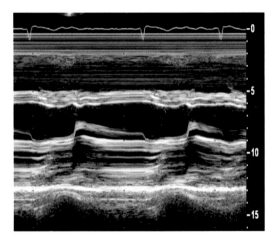

M-mode of Mitral Stenosis

The left ventricle M-mode of the interventricular septum may show a quick displacement posteriorly, as a result of right ventricular filling in early diastole at the expense of the left ventricle.

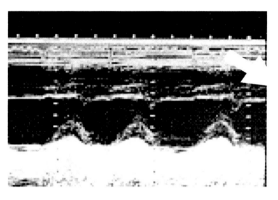

M-mode of IVS with Mitral Stenosis

Left atrial enlargement is typically noted on the M-mode exam. "Fuzzy" echoes may appear on the posterior aspect of the left atrium, but differentiation between artifact and clot is difficult due to location and size of the left atrium.

Two-Dimensional Study

The 2-D exam shows the visual extent of the involvement of the valve and its apparatus. An increase in echogenicity is variable depending on the amount of fibrotic and calcific changes. Chordal structures are thick, shortened and fibrotic. Diastolic doming or a "hockey stick" appearance may be noted on the anterior mitral leaflet as a result of the tethering of the leaflet tips.

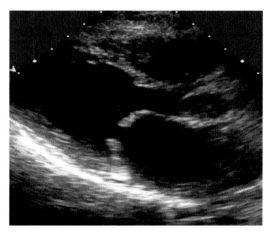

Doming of the MV leaflets from Mitral Stenosis

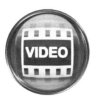

Play Video 3A: Parasternal Long Axis View of Mitral Stenosis

The left atrium is typically enlarged and can become quite dilated over time. As the left atrial size increases, the possibility of left atrial thrombus increases. Locating a left atrial thrombus may be difficult since left atrial clot often occurs in the left atrial appendage, an area not always well visualized on the transthoracic exam.

The best images for visualizing the LAA on TTE is in the PSA at the Aortic level and the Apical 2 chamber view. TEE is the exam of choice when there is a concern about a clot in the left atrial appendage.

Play Video 3B: LA Clot from Mitral Stenosis

The left ventricular size may be small to normal. The interventricular septum may show a momentary posterior displacement which is also noted on the M-mode exam. The left ventricle may be hypercontractile.

When pulmonary hypertension is present, the right atrial and ventricular size may be increased, and right ventricular hypertrophy may result. When the right side of the heart is enlarged, it is almost certain that tricuspid regurgitation will be present.

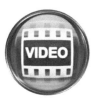

Play Video 3C: Apical 4 Chamber View of Mitral Stenosis

The mitral valve area may be measured on the 2-D examination in the short axis view. When the valve is at its maximum excursion, the orifice is planimetered. This event occurs at mid-diastole.

Planimetry should be performed on the inside edge of the leaflets if adequate visualization is possible. If diameter measurements are performed the equation to calculate mitral valve area is

MVA =1/2 transverse diameter x 1/2 vertical diameter x 3.14.

Excellent visualization of the mitral valve orifice is necessary to accurately calculate the mitral valve orifice using planimetry.

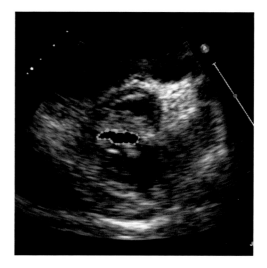

Planimetry of Mitral Valve Orifice

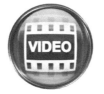

Play Video Clip 3D: PSAX mitral stenosis

Mitral Valve Area table:

Normal:	4- 6 cm²
Mild:	1.6 to 2-0 cm²
Moderate:	1.1 to 1.5 cm²
Severe:	1.0 cm² or less
Source: The Echo Manual (Oh et al.)	

Doppler Study

The Doppler evaluation of the mitral valve is imperative to give an accurate hemodynamic assessment of the severity of mitral stenosis. The normal flow through the mitral valve orifice should not be any greater than 1.5 m/s. High velocity flow is found distal to the obstruction and the best transducer position to perform the Doppler exam is the apical position.

A continuous wave Doppler transducer is necessary to obtain the most accurate flow velocities. Color flow imaging may be helpful in localizing the high velocity jet, typically displayed as a "candle flame" appearance. The continuous wave is directed towards the highest jet as indicated by the spectral tracing and audible changes in pitch. The Doppler tracing of mitral stenosis should be placed above the zero baseline and all aliasing of the signal corrected by adjusting the baseline and/or scale. The Doppler tracing demonstrates flattening of the wave and in severe cases an absence of the A wave. Spectral broadening is not always seen in cases of mitral stenosis.

Several calculations can be used to confirm the severity of the disease. Typically, the pressure half- time and mean pressure gradients show the most significant changes in patients with MS. The peak pressure gradient may also be obtained.

The pressure half-time is defined as the time in milliseconds it takes the mitral valve pressure gradient to drop to one-half of the original maximum peak transmitted pressure gradient. The longer it takes to reach ½ of the original, the more severe the stenosis.

A formula based on the pressure half-time (PHT) and Gorlin valve area has been derived to calculate mitral valve area.

Mitral Valve Area = $\dfrac{220}{PHT}$

The pressure half-time is calculated by measuring the mitral valve spectral tracing deceleration slope. Pressure half-times of less than 60 milliseconds are normal. A pressure half-time of 220 milliseconds is equivalent to a mitral valve area of approximately $1 cm^2$. Pressure half-time may be influenced by stroke volume, left ventricle diastolic compliance, tachycardia, first degree AV block, atrial flutter, and severe aortic regurgitation.

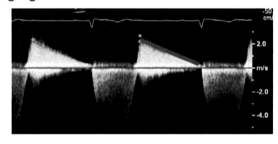

Pressure Half-time calculation of the MV

Peak and mean pressure gradients should also be calculated. Peak pressure gradients are determined by obtaining the peak mitral valve stenosis velocity and utilizing the modified Bernoulli equation, $4V^2$ where V is the peak velocity. Mean pressure gradients are performed by planimetering the stenotic valve envelope of the spectral tracing. The VTI, velocity time integral, also referred to as a TVI, or time velocity integral measures all the velocities in the envelope to give a mean velocity reading. Mean pressure gradients of 10 mmHg. or greater indicate severe stenosis, but pressure gradients are dependent on volume flow rate, as well as valve area.

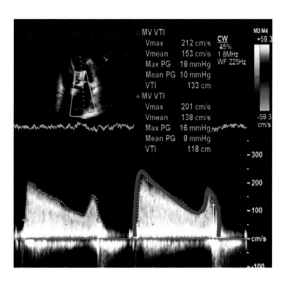

Mitral Stenosis VTI or TVI

Mean PG Values for the MV

Mild:	< 5 mmHg
Moderate:	5 – 10 mmHg
Severe:	> 10 mmHg
Source: The Echocardiographer's Pocket Reference, (Reynolds)	

The **continuity equation** should also be utilized as a method to determine the severity of mitral stenosis. The stroke volume from the LVOT diameter and VTI(TVI) and the VTI (TVI) of the mitral valve are required.

MVA = LVOT D² X 0.785 X VTI (LVOT) / VTI (MV)

The **PISA** method utilizes color flow imaging information to determine mitral valve area. PISA stands for proximal isovelocity surface area. The proximal isovelocity surface area is contained within the two mitral leaflets.

PISA = a/180 X hemispheric area.

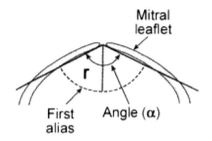

$$MVA\ cm^2 = \frac{6.28 \times r^2 \times Alias\ Velocity}{Peak\ mitral\ stenosis\ Velocity} \times \frac{a^o}{180^o}$$

All calculations are dependent on other factors in the heart. A prolonged pressure half-time may be seen on patients with abnormal myocardial relaxation. Patients with atrial fibrillation have hemodynamic variables so Doppler tracings from five to ten cardiac cycles should be used and an average taken. When the deceleration slope measurements vary on the mitral velocity, the pressure half-time should be obtained from the slope that has the longest duration. The pressure half-time measurement may be shortened when aortic valve regurgitation is present, resulting in an underestimation of mitral stenosis due to the rise in left ventricular end-diastolic pressure. The continuity equation may overestimate the severity of mitral stenosis when mitral regurgitation is present.

Patients with low cardiac output will have lower peak and mean pressure gradients that do not necessary reflect the severity of mitral stenosis.

Doppler should also be performed to evaluate for regurgitation in all of the valves and any other possible coexisting lesions.

Mitral Regurgitation

Mitral regurgitation is also referred to as mitral insufficiency. Mitral regurgitation is leakage of blood back into the left atrium due to some type of valve dysfunction. There are several etiologies causing mitral regurgitation. Many involve the valve leaflets, however, abnormalities of the other valve structures such as the muscle or chordal structures can also result in regurgitation.

Signs and symptoms of mitral regurgitation include: fatigue, dyspnea on exertion, angina, palpitations, orthopnea, edema, heart failure and right heart failure. During auscultation a high pitched blowing holosystolic murmur best heard at the cardiac apex and radiating to the axilla may be heard.

Mitral valve prolapse is the most common lesion causing mitral regurgitation. Mitral valve prolapse is a condition in which one or both leaflets of the mitral valve prolapse or sag into the left atrium. This condition is often a result of increased size and redundancy of one or both leaflets. The chordae can be elongated and the mitral ring is enlarged. Other terms used when referring to mitral valve prolapse are billowing mitral valve, floppy mitral valve, and Barlow's syndrome. Clinical indications of mitral valve prolapse with auscultation may be a mid-systolic click, a late systolic murmur, or a mid-systolic click followed by a late systolic murmur.

The patient may be asymptomatic or may complain of non-anginal chest pain, palpitations, dyspnea, and fatigue depending on the severity of the condition.

There are several mechanisms that can cause mitral valve prolapse. Three origins of the disease are usually considered: valvular, myocardial, and ischemic. Valvular origins of mitral valve prolapse may be a result of redundancy and or myxomatous degeneration of the leaflets. This often occurs in the anterior leaflet since it makes up 2/3 of the circumference of the mitral valve orifice. Myxomatous degeneration is a condition that is histologically characterized by disarray of the mitral leaflet, thickening, and an increase of mucopolysaccharides within the leaflet tissue, replacing normal tissue. Myxomatous degeneration may be a part of normal aging, but is also seen in younger patients. Another cause of valvular origin mitral valve prolapse is disparity in growth of the left ventricle compared to the mitral valve. This may be the reason why many young females with less body growth after puberty may have a smaller ventricle as compared to the annular circumference.

Myocardial factors may result in mitral valve prolapse. This may be caused by asymmetric ventricular contractions, a hyperkinetic left ventricle, or a hypokinetic left ventricle as seen in some cardiomyopathies. Displacement of the papillary muscles may also be a factor. Ischemic heart disease may result in papillary muscle dysfunction causing mitral valve prolapse.

The diagnosis of mitral valve prolapse with echocardiography is sometimes difficult. On the 2-D exam the parasternal long axis view is considered the best view in evaluation for mitral valve prolapse. Because the mitral valve annulus is saddle shaped, the valve appears to bow in the apical four chamber projection.

Mitral valve prolapse is diagnosed on the 2-D exam when one or both of the leaflets are displaced into the left atrium past the mitral valve annulus during systole. The leaflets may appear thick and redundant. Left atrial enlargement may be present depending on the severity of the disease. Aortic and tricuspid valve involvement may be seen on patients with myxomatous mitral valve disease.

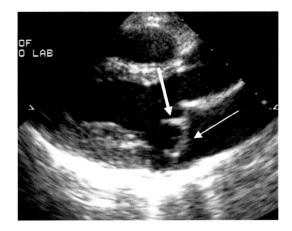

Mitral Valve Prolapse Parasternal Long

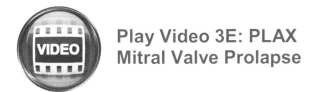

Play Video 3E: PLAX Mitral Valve Prolapse

M-mode consideration of mitral valve prolapse is made when the leaflet or leaflets are displaced posteriorly greater than 3 mm below the C-D points on the M-mode tracing of the valve. There may be some abnormal left ventricular posterior wall motion. Thickened leaflets, and left atrial enlargement may also be present.

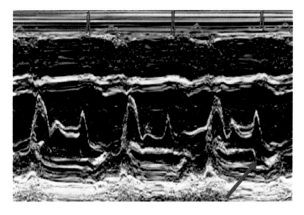

M-mode Mitral Valve Prolapse

Doppler findings are usually consistent with mitral regurgitation. Regurgitant jets may be eccentric so multiple views must be employed. An eccentric jet is usually seen opposite of the abnormal leaflet. Approximately 1/3 of mitral valve prolapse patients have mitral regurgitation. Approximately 1/3 of these patients also have a tricuspid valve prolapse. The jet is usually directed away from the prolapsing leaflet.

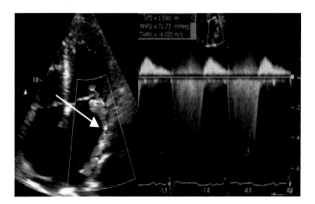

Eccentric Jet of Mitral Regurgitation

Mitral annular calcification may also result in mitral regurgitation. Calcification of the mitral annulus is often seen in elderly patients but is also seen in younger patients with mitral valve prolapse, renal failure and hypertension. Calcifications of the annulus range from small, to large and dense. They appear as areas of increased echogenicity on the left ventricular side of the annulus adjacent to the attachment point of the posterior leaflet.

The short axis view may best identify the extent of calcification, commonly appearing as a U-shaped area on the annulus. Shadowing is often seen as a result of the dense calcification causing impedance of the sound waves. Annular calcifications impair systolic contraction of the annulus that may result in mitral regurgitation. Up to 50% of patients with annular calcifications have mitral regurgitation. Often times calcifications of the aortic cusps are also noted. Clinically, these patients may have arrhythmias such as atrial fibrillation or premature beats.

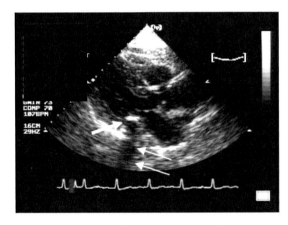

Mitral Annulus Calcification Parasternal Long Axis

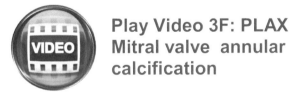

Play Video 3F: PLAX Mitral valve annular calcification

On the M-mode exam, annular calcifications appear as dense areas posterior to the mitral valve. This may have the appearance of fluid posterior to the valve due to the echo drop out. Often times the endocardium is not visualized due to the calcific nature.

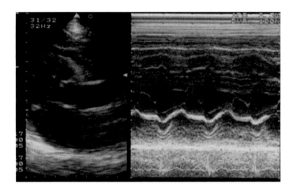

Mitral Annulus Calcification M-mode

Rupture of the chordae tendineae

may be responsible for a large number of patients with acute mitral regurgitation. Clinical symptoms include sudden onset of dyspnea that progresses quickly and chest pain suggesting myocardial ischemia. The patient typically develops heart failure. Rupture of the chordae does not always result in acute, severe mitral regurgitation. Isolated chordae ruptures or rupture of a non-critical chordae may result in intermittent chest pain, dyspnea, and mild pulmonary edema. Sometimes these symptoms mimic symptoms of pulmonary embolism or myocardial infarction.

Chordal rupture results from either abnormal stress on the chordae or a process that produces dysplasia and necrosis of the chordae. The normal chordae tether the mitral valve in early systole preventing prolapse of the leaflet. When this is altered the tension on the chordae is increased. Diseases that may affect the chordae are rheumatic endocarditis, Marfan's syndrome, idiopathic mitral valve prolapse, papillary muscle ruptures, and endocarditis.

Less common causes of chordal rupture are seen in patients with HOCM, trauma, non-bacterial endocarditis, achondroplasia with a coexistent atrial septal defect, aortic regurgitation, and patients with Ehlers- Danlos syndrome, an inherited disorder of the elastic connective tissue. Often times patients with spontaneous chordal rupture are noted to have abnormalities in elastin and collagen. Posterior leaflet chordae are thinner and more susceptible to rupture. Patients with spontaneous chordal rupture seem to commonly have rupture of the posterior leaflet and chordae suggesting there is more stress on this structure. When rupture is acute, surgical intervention may be required.

A mitral valve ring or Carpentier ring may be used to repair the valve.
The 2-D exam demonstrates a loss of leaflet coaptation. This may have what is referred to as a *"snake tongue"* effect. The mitral valve leaflet becomes **flail**. The chordae may be noted in the left atrium during systole. The affected leaflet tip will point into the left atrium and the left atrium may be enlarged.
The atrial septum may bend or bow towards the right atrium due to the increased left atrial pressure. The left ventricle will demonstrate hyperkinetic function.

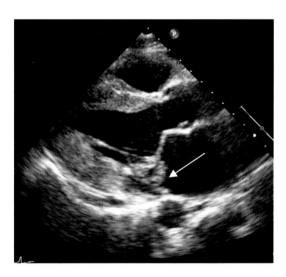

Flail Posterior Mitral Valve Leaflet

On the M-mode exam systolic fluttering of the leaflets may be noted. Left atrial enlargement and a hyperkinetic left ventricle will be noted. A mitral valve prolapse may be seen as well as erratic motion of the affected leaflet. The mitral leaflet may contact the interventricular septum due to increased diastolic excursion of the leaflet.

The Doppler exam will demonstrate moderate to severe regurgitation. On color flow imaging an eccentric jet will be seen opposite the flail leaflet.

<u>Papillary muscle dysfunction</u> is another cause of mitral regurgitation. There are several causes of papillary muscle dysfunction. They are ischemia, left ventricular dilatation, atrophy of the papillary muscle, defective development of the papillary muscles, endomyocardial disease, heart muscle disease, cardiomyopathy, and rupture of the papillary muscle. The most common of these causes is coronary artery disease.

Clinical symptoms may be angina, shortness of breath, and chest discomfort depending on the degree of mitral regurgitation and ischemia. A complication of papillary muscle dysfunction is papillary muscle rupture. Ischemia is the most common cause of papillary muscle dysfunction/rupture, but trauma may also cause a ruptured papillary muscle. Chances of survival are low when severe, acute mitral regurgitation results from a traumatic rupture because of the unstable hemodynamics.

On a 2-D exam, the ruptured papillary muscle appears as a mass attached to the flail segment of the mitral leaflet. The ruptured head of the muscle may be visualized in the left atrium and ventricle during systole and diastole. A partial rupture of the papillary muscle head may occur. This is the more common situation and may appear on the exam as a thin, attenuated, very mobile muscle.

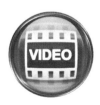

Play Video 3G & H: TEE of flail Mitral Valve leaflet from ruptured papillary muscle in Color and B&W

When mitral regurgitation is acute, the heart is ejecting blood both through the aorta, against systemic vascular resistance, and back into the left atrium which is low resistance. The effect on the left ventricle is a more efficient ejection of left ventricular blood resulting in an increased ejection fraction. The left ventricle does not dilate and the left ventricle becomes hyperdynamic.

When regurgitation is chronic, the left ventricle will dilate resulting in an increased left ventricular stroke volume. The left atrium will dilate to accommodate the regurgitant flow while keeping normal left atrial pressures. The left atrial compliance increases. This is not so in acute mitral regurgitation whereas the left atrium is non-compliant causing a significantly increased left atrial pressure without compensatory chamber dilation.

The increased left atrial pressure may cause a V wave on the left atrial pressure curve. As a result of increased left atrial pressures, either through chronic mild elevation and severe elevation with acute mitral regurgitation, the pulmonary artery pressure rises passively.

The pulmonary artery pressure can be estimated by obtaining the peak velocity of tricuspid valve regurgitation and applying that number to the Bernoulli equation. A factor of 5 or possibly higher is added as the assumed right atrial pressure depending on the size and collapsibility of the inferior vena cava. If the IVC is normal in size (< 2.1 cm) and collapses more than 50% with inspiration, the RA pressure is assumed to be 0 – 5 mmHG. If the IVC is normal in size but does not collapses more than 50%, the RA pressure is assumed to be 5 - 10 mmHG. However, if the IVC is dilated and fixed with inspiration, the RA pressure is assumed to be 15mmHG. For registry purposes, a standard 5 or 10 may be used.

(A more extensive discussion is provided under pulmonary hypertension.)

RVSP = 4V² + 10.
(15 may be added if higher RA pressure is suspected).

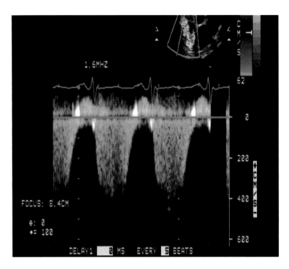

Tricuspid Regurgitation

The M-mode appearance of mitral regurgitation may include an increased left atrial size and increased motion of the aortic root.

The severity of mitral regurgitation may be evaluated by several methods on the Doppler exam. Continuous, pulsed, or color flow Doppler may be used. Multiple tomographic views are used from the apical position to evaluate mitral regurgitation.

90

A technical pitfall is the depth of the left atrium making complete evaluation of the mitral regurgitation sometimes difficult. Several methods of grading the severity of regurgitation have been suggested. The height, width and depth of the jet should be considered.

Doppler and color flow imaging methods may include measuring the area of the mitral regurgitation jet (regurgitant jet area) or by comparing the MR jet area to the area of the left atrium (regurgitant jet area over the left atrial area).

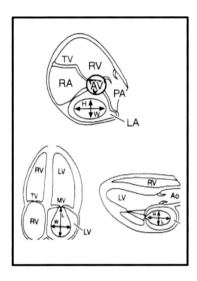

Jet Area/ Left Atrial Size

RJA/LAA and RJA	
Mild	<20%
Moderate	20 – 40%
Severe	>40%
RJA	
Mild	<4cm2
Moderate	4 – 8 cm2
Severe	> 8 cm2

Source: The Echocardiographer's Pocket Reference, (Reynolds)

Systolic flow reversal can be noted in the pulmonary veins as a result of the displacement of the left atrial blood by the regurgitant blood in severe mitral regurgitation. A false negative assessment of severe regurgitation occurs when the left atrium is chronically and severely enlarged leaving it compliant enough to contain all of the mitral regurgitation.

An eccentric jet may cause the appearance of pulmonary vein flow reversal without a severe degree of regurgitation resulting in a false positive assessment of severe regurgitation

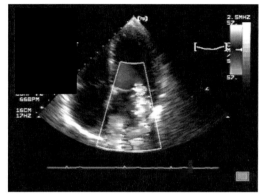

Mitral Regurgitation Into Pulmonary Vein

The intensity of the Doppler signal is an indication of the severity of mitral regurgitation. A well stained, well defined, high velocity signal with a continuous wave Doppler may be suggestive of severe regurgitation. In cases of chronic regurgitation, a continuous wave spectral recording indicates a quick rise in velocity from the baseline during isovolumetric contraction proportional to the rise of the left ventricle pressure. This is the dP/dt. The peak velocity is 5-6 m/s and velocities remain increased through all of systole. This flow curve parallels the left ventricle pressure with a normal left atrial pressure. The Doppler signal returns to the baseline quickly with isovolumetric relaxation.

When acute mitral regurgitation is present, there is a rise in left atrial pressure late in systole. The Doppler pattern has a V wave as a result of the steep pressure-volume relationship caused by the normal sized left atrium.

The left ventricle/left atrial pressure starts out high, but equalizes in late systole causing a high velocity signal initially, with a rapid fall in the middle of systole. The stroke volume of the mitral regurgitation can be calculated.

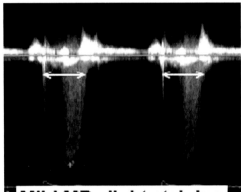

Mild MR - light staining

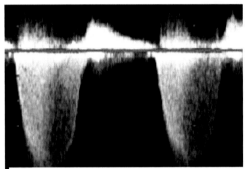

Severe MR - dark staining

Calculation of SV via MR

Mitral Regurg Volume	= Transmitral SV - Transaortic SV

The transmitral stroke volume is derived by obtaining the mitral valve annulus diameter and the velocity time integral of the flow across the annulus. The transaortic stroke volume is derived by obtaining the cross-sectional area and velocity time integral of the left ventricular outflow tract and flow.

This calculation is also referred to as the **Regurgitant Fraction method** and is useful because the result is a volume in cc's which is helpful when quantifying the severity of mitral regurgitation. This method cannot be employed with patients who have more than mild aortic insufficiency.

The PISA method may be employed to determine the severity of mitral regurgitation. Using color flow imaging, the proximal isovelocity surface area in the left ventricle can be identified.

Flow rate at PISA = Flow rate across regurgitant orifice.

Several steps are necessary to obtain the PISA. This method has been simplified and the regurgitant volume can be determined using the following equation:

$$MRV = 2 \times r^2 \times v$$

The ERO or effective regurgitant orifice can be determined by the following equation.

$$0.38 \times r^2 = ERO$$

Indications of severe mitral regurgitation are:
- ERO ≥ 0.40 cm²
- Mitral regurgitation volume > 60 cc's.

Other findings that are suggestive of severe mitral regurgitation are:

- Eccentric jet that reaches posterior left atrial wall.
- Color flow area ≥ 40% of the left atrium.
- E velocity ≥1.5m/s (> 2m/s prosthetic valves).
- Left ventricle dimension ≥ 7cm
- Left atrium ≥ 5.5cm
- Systolic reversal in pulmonary veins
- Vena contracta width ≥ 0.7 cm

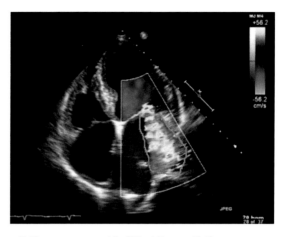

RJA measurement in Mitral Regurgitation

Mixed lesions of mitral stenosis and mitral regurgitation are important to evaluate to determine the predominant lesion. If the mitral valve area is less than 1.0 to 1.5 cm², mitral stenosis is the major hemodynamic lesion and the left ventricle should not have any significant volume loading. If the mitral valve orifice is greater than 2.0 cm², the mitral regurgitation is probably the predominant lesion. The left ventricle will have increased volume loading which is accentuated during early and mid-diastole.

When the mitral valve is fixed and immobile, but with an orifice of 1.5 to 2.0 cm², there may be some left ventricular volume overload and mitral stenosis, however, this is fairly uncommon.

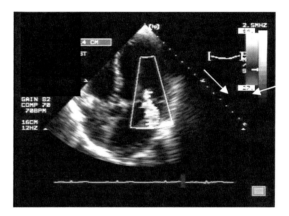

CFI to obtain ERO

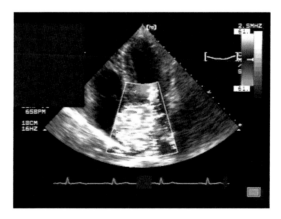

Severe Mitral Regurgitation / CFI

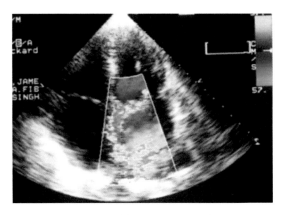

Eccentric Jet of Mitral Regurgitation

Classification of MR severity

MR	Mild	Severe
Jet area(cm^2)	<4	>8
JA/LAA(%)	<20	>40
Vena contracta (cm)	<0.3	>0.7
PISA (cm)	<0.4	>0.9
Regurg vol (ml)	<30	>60
Regurg fract (%)	<30	>50
ERO area (cm^2)	<0.20	>0.40

Source: The Echocardiographer's Pocket Reference (Reynolds)

AORTIC VALVE

Physiology & Hemodynamics

The aortic valve is a semilunar valve that regulates blood flow between the left ventricle and the ascending aorta. It is normally open during systole due to increased pressure from contraction of the left ventricle and at end systole when the pressure is much lower in the ventricle the aortic valve closes and should remain closed throughout diastole There is a short interval from when the mitral valve closes and before the aortic valve opens called *isovolumetric contraction time or IVCT.* In addition, there is a similar interval between the closure of the aortic valve and before the mitral valve opening called *isovolumetric relaxation time or IVRT.*

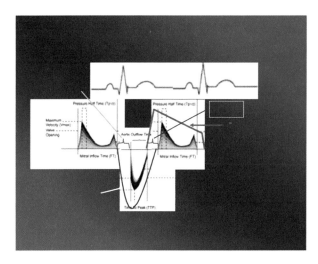

Diagram of Atrioventricular and Semilunar valve waveforms and timing

The flow across a semilunar valve, either the aortic valve or pulmonic valve, is parabolic in shape and corresponds to the building of pressure from contraction of the left and right ventricles respectively. This pattern is distinct from the biphasic diastolic pattern of the atrioventricular valves and is also in the opposite direction as noted in the previous diagram.

This diagram also illustrates the intervals of IVCT & IVRT with respect to the semilunar and atrioventricular valves. In addition, these intervals help determine if the flow obtained is from a normal semilunar valve or regurgitation from an incompetent atrioventricular valve based on the timing of the flow. This also works to differentiate stenotic high velocity flow from an AV valve versus regurgitant flow from an incompetent semilunar valve as shown.

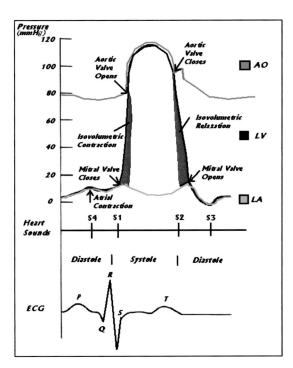

Diagram of Pressure changes & phases of systole

As was mentioned previously the aortic valve is a semilunar valve and it is similar to the pulmonic valve except its cusps are slightly thicker. The aortic valve has three fibrous cusps, the right, left, and non-coronary cusps. The cusps are suspended from the aortic root and are usually fairly equal in size. The sinuses of Valsalva lie behind each cusp and appears as pouch-like dilatations. The coronary arteries arise from the region of

95

the sinuses of Valsalva of the right and left coronary cusps.

Aortic Stenosis

Aortic stenosis is an abnormal narrowing of the valve orifice.

Aortic Valve Area

Normal	2-4 cm²
Mild stenosis	>1.5 cm²
Moderate stenosis:	1.0 – 1.5 cm²
Severe stenosis:	<1.0 cm².

Source: (The Echocardiographer's Pocket Reference, (Reynolds)

Stenosis of the valve orifice results in an increase in the velocity of blood flow across the valve correlating to an increase in the pressure gradient across the valve. If valve stenosis is isolated, symptoms usually begin to occur when the valve area is reduced to 1/4 of its normal size. The other cardiac chambers respond to valvular stenosis as well.

In the case of aortic stenosis, the left ventricle walls are hypertrophied or thickened due to the pressure overload, subsequently, the atria dilate in response. Any time valvular stenosis is encountered several parameters should be evaluated during the echocardiogram. Quantification of the severity of the stenosis with both 2-D and Doppler, determination and evaluation of other coexisting lesions, left ventricular function, and the response of upstream cardiac chambers and pulmonary vascular bed to chronic pressure overload should all be determined during the exam

Symptoms of aortic stenosis include chest pain, syncope, dyspnea, and congestive heart failure. Chest pain is the most common symptom. Syncope and near syncopal episodes are often noted with exertion and are not nearly as common as chest pain. Shortness of breath with left ventricular failure may be a symptom associated with both age

and physical exertion. During auscultation a harsh, systolic ejection murmur best heard at the second right intercostal space may be heard.

There are three types of aortic stenosis, congenital, rheumatic, and calcific or acquired. Congenital aortic stenosis is almost always a result of a unicuspid or bicuspid aortic valve. The bicuspid valve is the most common congenital malformation in the heart.

A **bicuspid valve** occurs in 1-2% of the population and is associated with coarctation of the aorta. **Coarctation** of the aorta is a localized narrowing resulting in a stricture often occurring in the aorta just past the level of the left subclavian artery take-off and ligamentum (ductus) arteriosus. Aortic stenosis occurring in patients before the age of 30 is usually the result of a unicuspid valve. A unicuspid valve may be non-commissural, but is often a unicommissural, domed valve.

A unicuspid valve usually has a single leaflet that begins at the aortic root wall and extends across the annulus, but does not contact the wall. The valve bends on itself and goes back to the wall and reattaches. The valve may have raphe, which is a crease or seam at the union of the two halves of the leaflet. A raphe may give the appearance of a bicuspid valve on a unicuspid valve and a tricuspid valve when a bicuspid valve is present. There is an inherent stenosis with a unicuspid valve and calcification develops on these valves at a young age. There is a 3:1 male over female predominance for unicuspid valves.

Bicuspid valves occur in 4 out of every 1,000 live births. There is a 4:1 predominance of males over females. Usually, leaflet thickening is present by the age of 30 or 40, but always by the age of 50. Calcification is rare before the age of 40, but by age 50 almost half have valve calcification.

Bicuspid valves are classified by two types. Type I, the cusps are located anteriorly and posteriorly with commissures on the left and right. Both coronary arteries will arise anterior to the anterior cusp. In type II the cusps are on the left and right and the commissures are anterior and posterior, and the coronary arteries arise from each cusp. One cusp may be large and contain a raphe, or they may both be equal in size. Bicuspid valves are not inherently stenotic like unicuspid valves, but the most common complication is stenosis. Regurgitation is the second most common complication. Damaged valves are also a nidus or cause for endocarditis, however, it has been noted that a heavily calcified bicuspid valve is rarely affected.

2-D findings of a bicuspid valve may demonstrate systolic bowing of the leaflets which appear dome-like on the long axis view. When the aortic valve is closed, a raphe can be confusing and may mimic the appearance of a normal tricuspid valve. Therefore, the determination of a bicuspid or unicuspid valve should be made when the valve is open during systole. The short axis view depicts a more oval type opening during systole rather than the usual triangular shaped opening of a normal tricuspid valve.

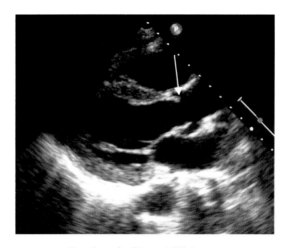

Doming of a Bicuspid Valve

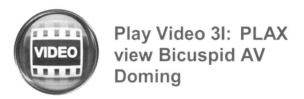

Play Video 3I: PLAX view Bicuspid AV Doming

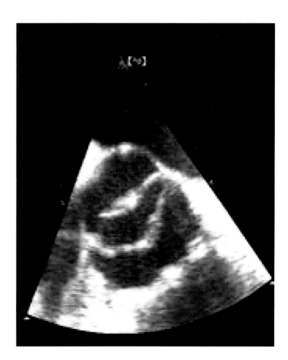

Short Axis of Bicuspid Valve During Systole

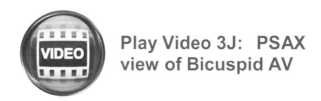

Play Video 3J: PSAX view of Bicuspid AV

The M-mode exam of a bicuspid valve commonly demonstrates eccentric closure of the valve. Eccentric closure is considered when valve closure is greater than 1/3 off from the midline of a normal aortic root.

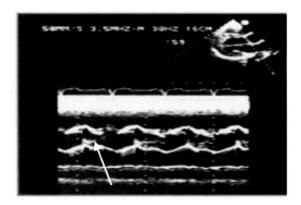

Mode Eccentric Closure Bicuspid Valve

Rheumatic valve disease usually
affects the mitral valve first. Often, aortic stenosis resulting from rheumatic valve disease is found during the evaluation for mitral stenosis when the aortic valve is at the early stages of the disease. When found in conjunction with mitral stenosis, aortic stenosis does not progress to more critical stages for 10 to 15 years. As with mitral stenosis, when aortic stenosis is a result of rheumatic disease; the commissures are fused. The 2-D exam may exhibit increased echogenicity along the edges of the cusps and systolic doming.

Calcific aortic stenosis is the most
common cause of aortic stenosis in adults. This calcific process occurs over years and may appear as sclerosis in the early stages.

Valvular sclerosis should be differentiated from stenosis. Sclerosis is a thickening or hardening of the tissue. A valve may have sclerotic changes that are a precursor to stenosis, but the valve orifice has not been affected

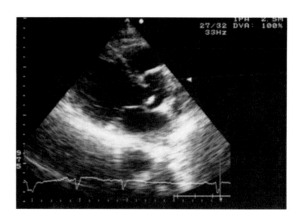

Aortic Valve Sclerosis Long Axis

Calcific aortic stenosis that results from aging does not typically become clinically significant until the patient is 70 - 85 years old. The appearance of calcified aortic stenosis is similar to that of aortic stenosis that is rheumatic in origin. The 2-D exam demonstrates the calcific areas that are usually seen at the base of the cusp and associated with reduced valve excursion. Systolic leaflet separation of less than 15mm suggests some degree of aortic stenosis. 2-D and M-mode determination of the aortic valve area can be very inaccurate so Doppler quantification should be employed. Additional findings with aortic stenosis are: left ventricular hypertrophy, left atrial enlargement, post stenotic dilatation of the aortic root, and irreversible changes in the other upstream chambers including the pulmonary vascular bed.

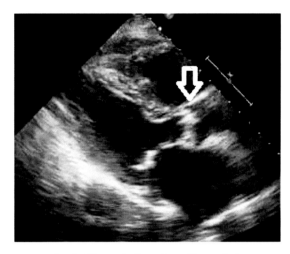

Aortic Stenosis Parasternal Long Axis

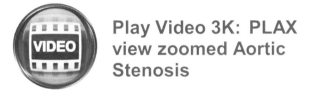

Play Video 3K: PLAX view zoomed Aortic Stenosis

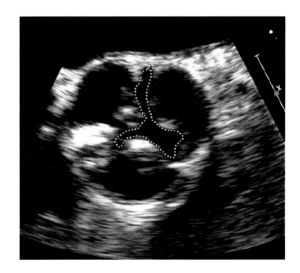

Aortic Stenosis Parasternal Short Axis

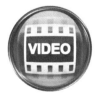

Play Video 3L: PSAX view zoomed Aortic Stenosis

M-Mode echocardiography demonstrates aortic stenosis with thick, dense echoes within the aortic root and aortic cusps excursion usually less than 15mm. The cusp excursion may not be identified due to the dense echoes within the root. The left ventricle typically hypertrophies with severe aortic stenosis or moderate, long standing disease. Left ventricular diameter may increase. Often times the left ventricle will be hypercontractile, but left ventricular function may decrease in a decompensated condition. The mitral valve E-F slope may become decreased as a result of the change in the left ventricular compliance.

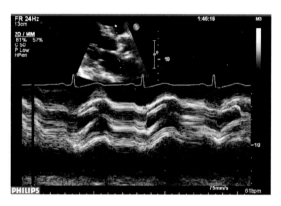

M-mode Calcific Aortic Stenosis

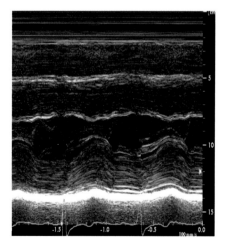

M-mode Left Ventricular Hypertrophy

The Doppler exam is often most helpful in the determination of the aortic valve area. Several quantification methods may be used. As stated previously, in

99

any stenotic valve, the peak pressure gradient can be easily calculated by obtaining the peak velocity of the stenotic lesion and applying it to the modified Bernoulli equation of:

$$\Delta P = 4V^2$$

Normal flow through all the valves is approximately 1 to 1.5 m/s, except for the tricuspid valve which is slightly less.

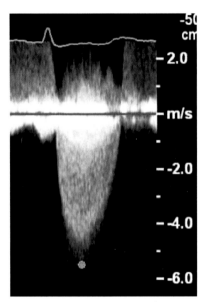

Doppler Peak Velocity Measurement

$$P = 4V^2$$
$$= 4 (5.25m/s)^2$$
$$= 110 \text{ mmHg}$$

Mean pressure gradients are calculated by averaging the instantaneous gradients over the systolic ejection period. This is done by tracing the stenotic jet envelope and is referred to as the VTI, or TVI.

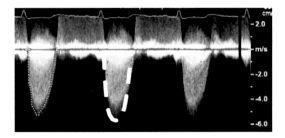

VTI or TVI (mean pressure gradient)

The aortic valve area can be estimated utilizing the **continuity equation**.

$$AVA = D^2 \text{ X } 0.725 \text{ X } \frac{\text{VTI LVOT (PW)}}{\text{VTI AoV (CW)}}$$

$$= \frac{SV}{TVI \text{ AoV}}$$

Measurement of the left ventricular outflow tract diameter, left ventricular outflow tract flow, and the highest velocity jet of flow distal to the stenosis must be obtained to perform the continuity equation.

The left ventricular outflow tract area is measured by obtaining a 2-D picture of the aortic valve in a parasternal long axis view and measuring the diameter of the left ventricular outflow tract at the site of cusp insertion into the walls. This measurement should be obtained at early systole right as the cusps separate.

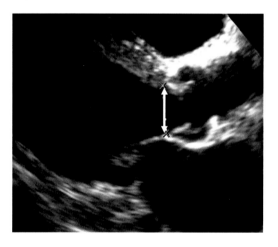

LVOT Diameter Measurement made in early systole

The left ventricular outflow velocity is found proximal to the aortic valve just before the valve with the **pulsed Doppler.** Sampling should be at the same level as the two-dimensional LVOT diameter.

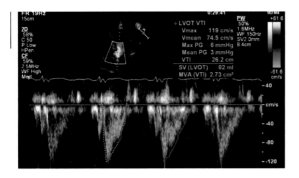

**LVOT Velocity Time Integral (VTI) or
Time Velocity Integral (TVI)**

The last step is to obtain the peak ascending aortic flow velocity. This can be done in the apical, right parasternal, or suprasternal positions using a **continuous wave Doppler transducer.**

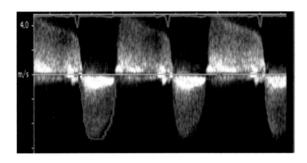

Aortic Velocity Time Integral (VTI) or TVI

Either a VTI / TVI measurement or peak velocity measurement may be utilized for the continuity equation to calculate aortic valve area. The VTI method does provides a mean pressure gradient which the peak velocity technique does not and this value may be required or preferred by some clinicians

The ASE recommends utilizing a "blind, non-imaging" PEDOF CW transducer to ensure obtaining the highest velocity from the stenotic jet

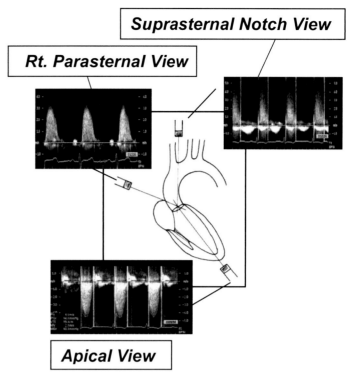

Rt. Parasternal View

Suprasternal Notch View

Apical View

DOPPLER VIEWS FOR AORTIC STENOSIS USING PEDOF PROBE

Due to potential jet eccentricity (see the following diagram) all the various sites should be interrogated to acquire the highest velocity waveform.

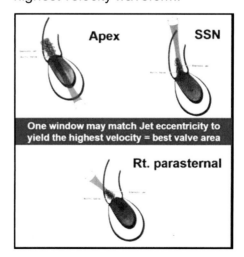

PEDOF CW probe windows for Aortic Stenosis

Failure to obtain the highest actual velocity could result in underestimation of the severity of stenosis by over estimating the aortic valve area.

Pitfalls to these measurements typically are technical in nature. Calcified valves make measuring the left ventricular outflow tract difficult and eccentric jets of aortic stenosis may be missed or technically difficult to obtain. Color flow imaging may be helpful in locating the eccentric jets.

Estimation of cardiac output

Cardiac output = SV x HR = L/min

The following four criteria are suggested for severe aortic stenosis in patients with otherwise normal left ventricular systolic function and cardiac output.

Criteria for Severe Aortic Stenosis

Mixed lesions of aortic stenosis and aortic regurgitation may cause increased transaortic pressure gradients due to increased transaortic volume flow. This should not affect calculations since the stroke volume in the continuity equation is the transaortic stroke volume. Patients with mitral stenosis and aortic stenosis may have lower transaortic pressure gradients due to the decreased volume flow. This leads to a falsely decreased determination of aortic valve area.

Females and males may respond differently to aortic stenosis. Females have a tendency to have small, hypertrophied left ventricles with normal systolic function, but males have less left ventricular hypertrophy and more left ventricular dilatation with a high incidence of left ventricular dysfunction.

Aortic Regurgitation

There are several etiologies for aortic regurgitation or insufficiency. Regardless of the cause, either an abnormality of the aortic root or the aortic cusps is present. As previously discussed, causes of aortic stenosis are also possible causes of aortic regurgitation. These include bicuspid and unicuspid valve, calcific valve disease, and rheumatic valve disease. There are other causes of regurgitant aortic valve disease, but without concomitant stenosis. Until the widespread use of prophylactic antibiotics, rheumatic fever and syphilis were the most common causes of aortic valve disease. Syphilitic aortitis is now rare in the United States, but characterized by a dilated aortic root with extensive calcification.

Myxomatous valve disease, also a cause of mitral regurgitation, can affect the aortic valve. Myxomatous valve disease is a disorder of the connective tissue in which normal tissue is disrupted and replaced by abnormal tissue, resulting in valvular incompetence. Myxomatous valve disease is usually progressive. Leaflets may prolapse and displacement is noted in the left ventricular outflow tract during diastole. Mitral and tricuspid valve prolapse may be associated findings.

Endocarditis may be a cause of aortic regurgitation. Endocarditis is an inflammation of the valve or lining of the heart. When an already damaged valve is exposed to infection, the infection may spread to the cusps. This may cause the cusps to prolapse or become flail.

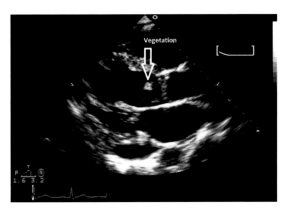

Parasternal Long Axis AV Endocarditis

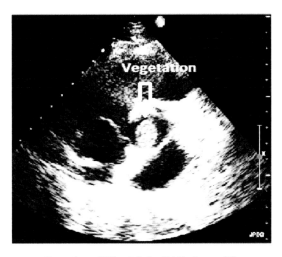

Parasternal Short Axis AV Endocarditis

Non-bacterial thrombotic endocarditis is a lesser cause of aortic regurgitation. This is a result of Libman-Sachs vegetations in patients with systemic lupus, infiltrative diseases such as amyloid, and collagen-vascular disorders.

Patients with **ankylosing spondylitis** may develop cardiovascular lesions. This is a progressive form of arthritis affecting men primarily. Greater than 90% of the people affected are in age range of 10 - 30. If the aortic valve is involved the lesions are located primarily in the areas above and below the aortic valve. Pathologic changes appear very similar to those with syphilitic aortitis. The regurgitation is a result of the thickening and shortening of the aortic cusps, dilation of the root, and cusp

displacement due to fibrous tissue that forms behind the commissures.

A small percentage of patients with **Reiter's syndrome** may develop aortic regurgitation. Reiter's syndrome also occurs mainly in young men and has an unknown etiology. The syndrome consists of urethritis, arthritis, and conjunctivitis. Aortic regurgitation usually occurs 15 years after the disease begins and results from the same pathologic changes as ankylosing spondylitis.

Patients with **rheumatoid arthritis** may develop aortic regurgitation as a result of focal valvular lesions. These lesions begin as a reaction within the center of the valve leaflet. This is different from rheumatic valve disease which affects the whole cusp. In these patients the mitral valve is usually involved first, followed by the aortic valve, tricuspid, and pulmonic valves respectively.

Some diseases affect the aortic root rather than the valve. These often cause dilation of the root preventing normal valve closure or coaptation.

Chronic hypertension is a common cause of aortic root dilatation. Other diseases causing aortic root dilatation are Marfan's' syndrome, cystic medial necrosis, and aortic dissection.

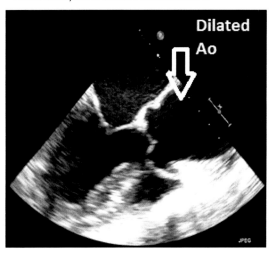

Ascending Aortic Aneurysm from TEE image

Marfan's syndrome is a hereditary disorder of the connective tissue, muscle, bones, ligaments, and skeletal structures. Cardiac involvement usually includes aortic root aneurysm typically at the level of the annulus, sinuses of Valsalva, and ascending aorta. The 2-D appearance may be termed the *"Water Balloon"* appearance. Associated findings include a long, redundant anterior mitral leaflet that sags into the left atrium during systole, and possible dissection.

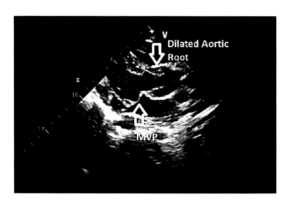

Parasternal Long Axis Marfan's Syndrome

Cystic medial necrosis is another disease causing aortic regurgitation. The elastic fibers of the arterial wall media are fragmented. This results in clefts filled with cystic deposits of mucoid material, typically affecting the ascending aorta, sometimes the pulmonary artery, and less often other large arteries. This process causes a weakening of the aortic root walls and subsequent dilation.

Aortic dissection can result in aortic regurgitation. A dissection is a tear in the intimal layer of the arterial wall, causing a false channel or lumen between the intima and media of the artery. The false lumen may expand causing compression of the true lumen. The dissection may continue throughout the aorta and its branches. Thrombus may also occur. There are several causes of aortic dissection. Patients with congenital bicuspid or unicuspid valves have a five times higher risk for dissection. Patients with pre-

existing aneurysms are also high risk. Chronic hypertension is the most common risk factor for dissection, however, atherosclerosis, and trauma are also possibilities. Aortic dissection can be a life threatening condition.

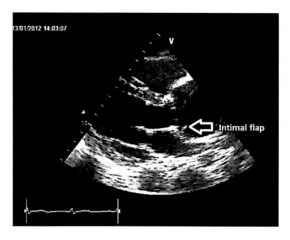

Aortic Dissection Showing Intimal Flap

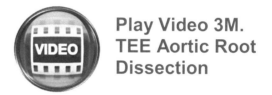

Play Video 3M. TEE Aortic Root Dissection

The valve should be evaluated to determine the anatomy and etiology of the regurgitation. The aortic root size should be measured and not exceed approximately 37 mm. The cusps are evaluated for number, thickening, and mobility. The left ventricle is evaluated for size and function along with any other associated abnormalities. The aortic regurgitant jet may impinge on the anterior mitral leaflet resulting in an increased EPSS due to leaflet flattening by the jet. The anterior mitral leaflet may have high frequency fluttering, typically appreciated on the M-mode exam. The anterior mitral leaflet may appear bowed due to the regurgitant jet and is sometimes referred to as reversed doming.

Patients with chronic regurgitation aimed towards the interventricular septum or the anterior mitral leaflet may have a raised, fibrotic lesion appearing as an area of increased echogenicity. This is referred to as a "jet lesion". The aortic regurgitant jet that is directed toward the anterior mitral valve leaflet can cause premature closure of the mitral valve during mid diastole which has been described as an *"Austin Flint"* murmur.

Play Video 3N: Apical 3 Chamber View of patient with "Austin Flint" murmur

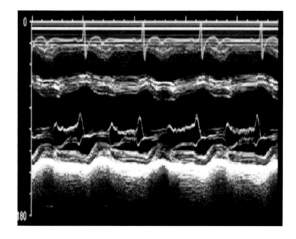

Fine fluttering of the Ant. MV with AI

Chronic aortic regurgitation usually results in a left ventricular volume overload and subsequent left ventricular dilation. The left ventricle has a spherical rather than conical appearance. Left ventricular function and left ventricular end diastolic pressures stay normal for a long time, but eventually the left ventricle will increase in size and systolic dysfunction occurs. A left ventricular diastolic dimension of 7.5 cm or greater may be seen with severe, chronic aortic regurgitation. The left ventricle is typically less than 6.0 cm with mild, chronic regurgitation.

Acute aortic regurgitation does not usually affect left ventricular size, but left ventricular end diastolic pressures are elevated. The left ventricle may be hyperdynamic. The atria are not usually affected unless left ventricular dysfunction occurs or other valvular problems are present.

The M-mode exam may show signs of aortic regurgitation. If the jet is directed towards the anterior mitral leaflet, then there may be an increased EPSS and fine fluttering of the anterior mitral leaflet. If the jet is directed towards the interventricular septum, the septum may flutter. The left ventricle may be enlarged with either normal or hyperdynamic function and left ventricular hypertrophy may be present.

The M-mode tracing of the mitral valve may have a "B" bump or notch indicating elevated left end diastolic pressures. The aortic valve may open prematurely when acute aortic regurgitation is present.

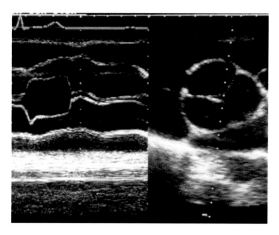

Aortic Insufficiency by M-mode and 2-D

Doppler assessment of aortic regurgitation helps to determine its severity. Pulsed mapping techniques have almost been completely replaced by color flow imaging to help define the length, width, and height of the jet. The short axis view on the color flow image may be the most helpful to tell the exact origin of the regurgitation. The left ventricular outflow height and the height of the regurgitant jet are obtained from the parasternal long axis view and the short axis view is used to obtain the regurgitant jet area.

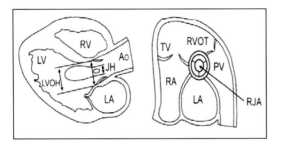

CFI Estimation of Aortic Regurgitation

Continuous wave Doppler indicates moderate to severe aortic regurgitation when the signal is easily recorded all through diastole and is well stained or dense. Aortic regurgitation is displayed above the zero baseline or displayed in red on color flow imaging. With moderate to severe regurgitation, the jet is holodiastolic. A steep deceleration slope may suggest chronic, severe regurgitation as the pressure gradient between the aorta and left ventricle is rapidly equalized. Using a pressure half-time calculation may give an indication of the severity of the regurgitation. A pressure half-time of less than 200 milliseconds suggests severe regurgitation.

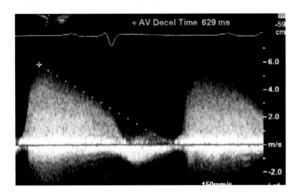

Pressure Half-Time Aortic Regurgitation

With acute aortic regurgitation, the Doppler signal may appear triangular shaped rather than the box-like

configuration seen with chronic aortic regurgitation. The shape of the aortic regurgitation velocity curve may also be affected by systolic dysfunction, ischemia, and aortic diastolic pressure. A shortened E velocity on the mitral valve deceleration time may give an indication of the severity of aortic regurgitation as a result of the decreased systemic diastolic pressure more typically associated with acute aortic regurgitation.

In cases of severe aortic regurgitation, holodiastolic flow reversal will be noted in the abdominal or thoracic aorta. This finding is analogous to diastolic reversal in the femoral arteries found on physical examination. The finding of diastolic reversal in the femoral arteries is referred to as DeRosier's Sign. A finding of holodiastolic flow reversal is 100% sensitive and 97% specific for the diagnosis of severe aortic regurgitation.

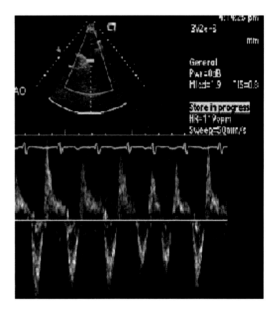

Holodiastolic Flow Reversal in the Descending Aorta

A false positive finding of holodiastolic flow reversal for aortic regurgitation may be seen in patients with patent ductus arteriosus or cerebral arteriovenous malformation`.

Other parameters used to determine the severity of aortic regurgitation are the aortic valve regurgitant volume which is the difference between the stroke volume across the left ventricular outflow tract and the mitral valve.

Ao Reg Vol. = LVOT flow – MV flow

= (D² X 0.785 X VTI) LVOT

– (Annulus D² X 0.785 X VTI) MV

The aortic regurgitant fraction may also be a helpful parameter or adjunct to the Doppler study.

RF = <u>Aortic Reg V</u>   X 100%
         LVOT stroke volume

ERO or the effective regurgitant orifice is another method to determine aortic regurgitation and is obtained by dividing the regurgitant volume by the aortic regurgitant TVI.

Often when aortic regurgitation and stenosis are found together, the regurgitation is the predominant lesion. Just as with mitral stenosis and regurgitation, when aortic stenosis and aortic regurgitation are concomitant, severe aortic stenosis is hemodynamically impossible if the aortic regurgitation is severe.

The following table lists several of the findings associated with *severe aortic regurgitation:*

Findings Associated with Severe Aortic Regurgitation

Regurgitant jet width/LVOT diameter ratio	≥ 60%
Regurgitant jet area/LVOT area ratio	≥ 60%
PHT (ao regurg)	≤200msec
Regurgitant fraction	≥ 55%
Regurgitant volume	≥60mL
ERO	≥0.30cm²
Vena contracta width	>0.6cm

Source: The Echo Manual (Oh et al.)

The following table lists several findings associated with *mild aortic regurgitation.*

Findings Associated with Mild Aortic Regurgitation

Regurgitant jet width/LVOT diameter ratio	≤ 30%
Regurgitant jet area/LVOT area ratio	≤ 30%
PHT (ao regurg)	≥500msec
Regurgitant fraction	< 30%
Regurgitant volume	≥60mL
ERO	< 0.10cm²
Vena contracta width	<0.3cm

Source: The Echo Manual (Oh et al.)

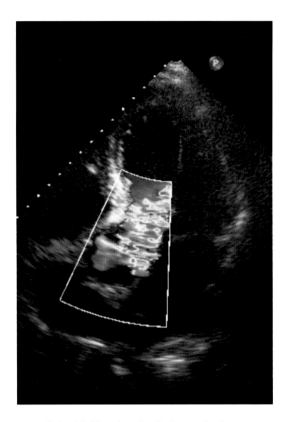

Apical 5 Chamber Aortic Regurgitation

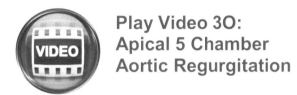

Play Video 3O:
Apical 5 Chamber
Aortic Regurgitation

TRICUSPID VALVE

Physiology and Hemodynamics

The tricuspid valve like the mitral valve is an atrioventricular valve. The tricuspid valve regulates blood flow from the right atria into the right ventricle Like the mitral valve, the normal tricuspid valve opens during diastole and closes during systole, but in this case, in response to changes in pressure between the right atrium and right ventricle. Although M-mode is seldom done on the tricuspid valve, it would have the same characteristic M shape as the mitral valve in response to the biphasic *early or rapid filling* phase and the *atrial contraction* phase of diastole.

Doppler interrogation is preferred for evaluation of the tricuspid valve. The Doppler waveform pattern is very similar to that of the mitral with an **E wave** and an **A wave** velocity but unlike the mitral which does not vary with respiration the **E wave** and **A wave** of the tricuspid valve will vary with deep inspiration. Another difference between the right and left side of the heart is the length of ventricular contraction which is typically longer for the right heart. Meaning that the tricuspid valve will open before the mitral valve opens and closes after the mitral valve closes. (See diagram labeled heart sounds and valve timing.)

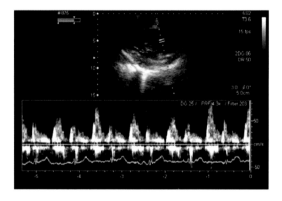

Tricuspid Inflow showing variation in E wave and A wave with respiration.

108

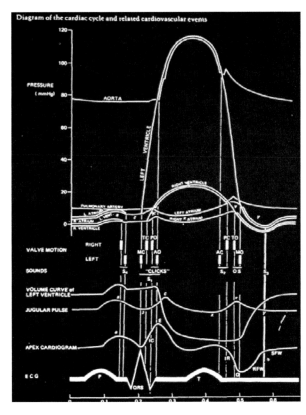

Diagram of heart sounds and valve timing

As previously mentioned, tricuspid valve is the right atrioventricular valve and has an orifice larger than the left atrioventricular valve, or mitral valve. Slightly more apically displaced than the mitral valve, it is somewhat anteriorly located below the left sternal border. The tricuspid leaflets are thinner than the mitral leaflets consisting of three, unequal in size leaflets, the septal or medial leaflet, the posterior leaflet, usually the smallest, and the anterior leaflet. The tricuspid valve directs blood flow anteriorly, inferiorly, and to the left from the right atrium to the right ventricle.

Tricuspid stenosis

The most common cause of acquired tricuspid stenosis is secondary to rheumatic valvulitis. To a much lesser degree, congenital heart disease, carcinoid heart disease, fibroelastosis, endomyocardial fibrosis, systemic lupus, and tumor obstruction are also causes.

When the tricuspid valve is affected by rheumatic valvulitis, there is commonly fusion of the adjacent free edges of the leaflets. This fusion causes a funnel-shaped structure. The anteroseptal commissures may be involved and the leaflets thicken moderately, but stay pliable. The chordae do not usually become severely deformed as with mitral stenosis and calcification of the valve is rare. Mitral stenosis almost always coexists with tricuspid stenosis when the origin of the tricuspid stenosis is rheumatic valvulitis.

The typical patient with tricuspid stenosis is a 20-48-year-old commonly presenting with a dominant coexisting lesion of mitral stenosis. The most common clinical pattern indicating tricuspid stenosis are patients complaining of effort intolerance and fatigue. Late stage clinical indications associated with tricuspid stenosis are fluttering in the neck due to venous distension and peripheral edema. The auscultatory feature that is characteristic of tricuspid stenosis is a mid-diastolic or pre-systolic murmur at the left sternal border in the fourth or fifth rib space. The murmur is timed relative to the cardiac rhythm. Carvallo's sign is a valuable ausculatory finding in tricuspid stenosis indicated by an increase in intensity of the diastolic murmur with inspiration.

Hemodynamically, the major problem with tricuspid stenosis is decreased cardiac output, increased venous distension and increased right atrial pressure. Severe tricuspid stenosis is present when the valve area is 1.0 cm² or less. The normal tricuspid valve area is greater than 7 cm². When tricuspid stenosis is present, the right atrium may enlarge, and atrial fibrillation can be present. The right ventricle may be normal or enlarged.

Carcinoid syndrome is another cause of tricuspid stenosis. Carcinoid syndrome results from metastatic tumors that secrete large amounts of vaso active substances. These substances include serotonin, bradykinin, histamine, and prostaglandins. The tumors usually originate from argentaffin cells in the intestinal tract, bile ducts, pancreas, bronchus, or ovaries.

Cardiac manifestations usually occur late in the syndrome. Hepatic metastasis is almost always associated, except when ovarian cancer is the primary. This is due mainly to the direct discharge of the ovarian endocrine product into the systemic venous circulation. The high amount of these vasoactive substances cause thickening of the valve and endocardium. The chordae become thickened, retracted, and fused, causing stenosis. It is also important to rule out the presence of a patent foramen ovale in these patients as left heart valves become involved in their presence.

Metastatic carcinoid lesions may be located in the myocardium. It is rare that the left side of the heart is involved. Clinically, patients with carcinoid disease may have flushing of the face and neck, tachycardia, edema of the face and periorbital region, hypotension, possible abdomen pain, diarrhea, weight loss, and hypoproteinemia. These symptoms usually develop after metastasis.

Tricuspid atresia is the absence of the usual flow orifice to the right ventricle. This leaves only the interatrial communication such as a patent foramen ovale for blood to pass from the right to left. Often there is an interventricular septal defect, allowing blood to pass from the left ventricle to the right ventricle and lungs. If there is not a ventricular septal defect the ductus arteriosus and bronchial arteries provide pulmonary circulation. Cyanosis is

probable and other cardiac defects may coexist.

Fibroelastosis is an overgrowth of fibroelastic tissue which can cause thickening and stenosis of the valve.

Endomyocardial fibrosis is rare in the United States. This heart disease is found in tropical countries, especially Africa, where it may account for up to approximately 10% of all cardiac disease. It usually affects older children and young adults. The endocardium is most often affected, but the myocardium and pericardium may be involved.

The onset of the disease typically starts with an acute onset of edema and breathlessness associated with fever. The pericardium is infiltrated by inflammatory cells and septal fibrosis tissue penetrates the myocardium from the endocardium. Lesions may occur in the ventricle outflow tracts, under the septal leaflet of the tricuspid valve, and the posterior mitral valve leaflet. Fibrotic tissue may line the ventricles causing cavity obliteration, bind papillary muscles, and cause the chordae to become adherent to the septum. Regurgitation and stenosis are possible consequences.

Tricuspid stenosis may be a result of **systemic lupus erythematosus**, a chronic disease of unknown cause. It is characterized by an autoimmune problem and is a systemic illness. Myocardial fibers, pericardial thickening, and constrictive pericarditis may result. Occasional valvular thickening occurs and more often causes mitral or aortic stenosis, but occasionally affects the tricuspid valve.

The 2-D exam of tricuspid stenosis is similar to that of mitral stenosis. The leaflets are thickened with reduced movement of the chordae and leaflets. Diastolic doming of the valve may be noted. Tricuspid annular calcification is not commonly found.

M-mode findings are limited due to the difficulty in obtaining tracings of the entire valve. Valve excursion is restricted and the E-F slope flattened as in mitral stenosis.

Doppler is the most accurate method of assessing tricuspid stenosis on the transthoracic echocardiogram. Color flow imaging demonstrates a "candle-flame" appearance as with mitral stenosis. Velocities are high and aliasing of flow is present. Peak velocities in tricuspid stenosis will be lower than those of mitral stenosis due to the large capacity of the venous bed. Peak velocities with tricuspid stenosis generally never exceed 1.8 m/s or gradients of 4-8 mmHg. These numbers are consistent with severe tricuspid stenosis, but not severe mitral stenosis. Tricuspid regurgitation may also be present.

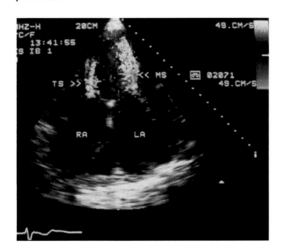

Color flow imaging of tricuspid and mitral stenosis with characteristic *"candle flame"* appearance

Tricuspid Regurgitation

Tricuspid regurgitation or insufficiency results from improper valve closure and subsequent leakage of blood into the right atrium. Due to the floppy nature of the tricuspid valve, there may be a small amount of physiologic regurgitation in patients with essentially a normal valve.

Clinical indications of significant tricuspid regurgitation includes right heart failure, a holosystolic murmur that may vary with respiration, and a third heart sound. In cases of severe tricuspid regurgitation, jugular venous distension is common, and right heart failure is possible.

Rheumatic valvulitis may cause thickening of the leaflets and commissural fusion. Rheumatic valve involvement occurs in approximately 20-30% of cases and almost always occurs in conjunction with mitral valve disease.

Carcinoid disease may also cause tricuspid regurgitation. As discussed previously, carcinoid disease is rare and usually seen with metastatic carcinoid tumors typically of the liver. The valve leaflets become shortened and immobile resulting in regurgitation.

Tricuspid valve prolapse occurs when the tricuspid leaflets may prolapse or bulge into the right atrium. Often, tricuspid valve prolapse is seen in conjunction with mitral valve prolapse.

Endocarditis may affect the tricuspid valve especially in cases of intravenous drug abuse. If vegetations occur on the valve leaflets, they may prolapse. In severe cases, the vegetations may destroy the valve apparatus causing the leaflet or leaflets to become flail. On the 2-D exam the leaflet points into the right atrium. Blunt force trauma to the chest may also cause flail leaflets due to chordal rupture.

Ebstein's anomaly is a congenital defect of the tricuspid valve. One or more of the valve leaflets are displaced from the annulus towards the apex. Usually the septal leaflet is involved with either the anterior or posterior leaflet. The degree of apical displacement is variable. Ebstein's anomaly is present when the separation between the mitral valve and the tricuspid valve is greater than 10mm.

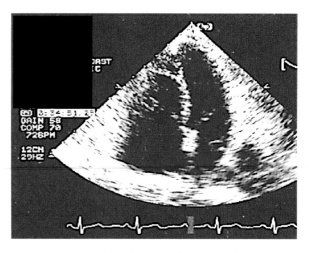

Dilated Right Atrium/Ventricle and RVH

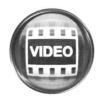

Play Video 3P: Patient with Ebstein's Anomaly

Pulmonary hypertension can cause tricuspid regurgitation. Pulmonary hypertension results when the pulmonary arterial pressures rise above normal, which is generally 35/15 mmHg. This pressure is dependent upon physiologic relationships between the volume of pulmonary arterial blood flow per unit of time and resistance to that flow. Factors responsible for this are elevation of pulmonary capillary and/or left atrial pressure, a decrease in cross-sectional area of the total pulmonary vascular bed, or a large increase in pulmonary arterial blood flow. There are other minor factors that may influence pulmonary artery pressure. When one or more of these situations occur, pulmonary hypertension may result. The 2-D exam of the right heart exhibits enlarged, hypertrophic right ventricle walls, and often times paradoxical septal motion. Tricuspid regurgitation results as a consequence of annular dilation.

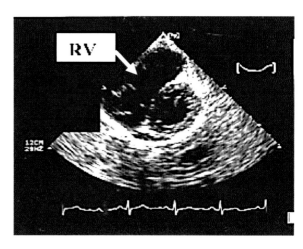

Enlarged Right Ventricle (Short Axis) Flattened IVS

M-mode findings for tricuspid regurgitation are non-specific. Right ventricular hypertrophy, right ventricular dilation, and septal paradoxical motion may be noted. Tricuspid prolapse or a prolonged A-C interval may also occur.

The Doppler assessment used on the mitral valve can be applied to the tricuspid valve in the evaluation of tricuspid regurgitation. In cases of severe tricuspid regurgitation, systolic flow reversal is noted in the hepatic veins. Color flow imaging shows tricuspid regurgitation in shades of blue in the right atrium with probable mosaic effects in high velocity jets. A well stained continuous wave signal may also suggest severe regurgitation. Chronic regurgitation has a rounded curve with peak velocities occurring in mid to late systole compared to the V shaped curve, early systolic peak velocities, and more rapid decline in late systole that is seen with acute tricuspid regurgitation.

Pulmonary artery pressure or **right ventricular systolic pressure** can

be measured by obtaining the peak velocity of the tricuspid regurgitation jet. This is done by assuming a right atrial pressure of 10mmHg.

RVSP = 4V²+ 5

A normal right ventricular systolic pressure is less than 35mmHg. A higher right atrial pressure can be assumed when the right atrium bulges towards the left atrium, the IVC and hepatic veins are dilated. This technique visualizes the IVC from the subcostal view at rest and during inspiration. The American Society of Echocardiography (ASE) recommends that the overall size of the IVC is noted at the point where it passes through the diaphragm and enters the right atrium and collapsibility with respiration is noted. If the IVC is dilated and does not collapse >50% with changes in respiration a higher right atrial pressure

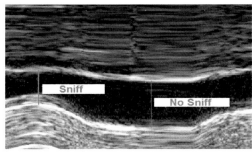

is suspected.

IVC Response indicating RA pressure is normal

American Society of Echocardiography recommends the following caval index:

	IVC size	Collapse	Est. RAP
Normal	<2.1cm	>50%	0-5mmHg
Intermediate	<2.1cm	<50%	5-
	>2.1cm	>50%	10mmHg
High	>2.1cm	<50%	15mmHg

Source: The Echocardiographer's Pocket Reference, (Reynolds)

Some authors recommend IVC diameters between 2.0 - 2.5 cm while other investigators suggest that caval diameter does not correlate as consistently as changes in collapsibility with respiration which they feel is much more reliable.

As with mitral regurgitation, severe tricuspid regurgitation should be suspected when the continuous wave Doppler signal is dense or well stained. Other indications of severe tricuspid regurgitation are dilation of the annulus 4cm or greater, increased velocity of the tricuspid inflow that is 1m/s or greater, late systolic concave configuration of the Doppler signal, and a color flow regurgitant jet area ratio to the right atrial area of 30% or greater.

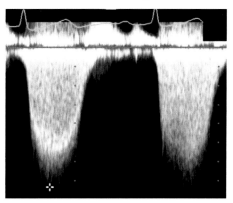

CW Tricuspid Regurgitation

Remember that pulmonary artery pressure or right ventricular systolic pressure severity does not indicate the severity of the regurgitation. There may be significant tricuspid regurgitation with a normal pulmonary artery pressure or mild to moderate tricuspid regurgitation with an elevated pulmonary artery pressure.

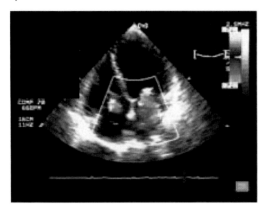

Mild Tricuspid/Moderate Mitral Regurgitation

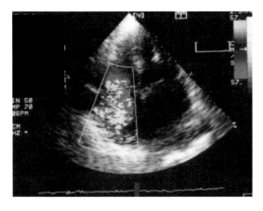

Severe Tricuspid Regurgitation

PULMONARY VALVE

Physiology and Hemodynamics

The pulmonary valve is a semilunar valve that regulates blood flow between the right ventricle and the pulmonary artery. It is normally open during systole due to increased pressure from contraction of the right ventricle and at end systole when the pressure is much lower in the ventricle the pulmonary valve closes and should remain closed throughout diastole.

The flow across this semilunar valve, much like the aortic valve, is parabolic in shape and corresponds to the building of pressure from contraction of the right ventricle. Again, this pattern is distinct from the biphasic diastolic pattern of the atrioventricular valves and is also in the opposite direction. *(See aortic valve for diagram demonstrating flow pattern of semilunar valves.)*

As with the tricuspid and mitral valves, the timing of events is slightly longer on the right side of the heart and therefore the pulmonic valve opens first and closes after the aortic valve.

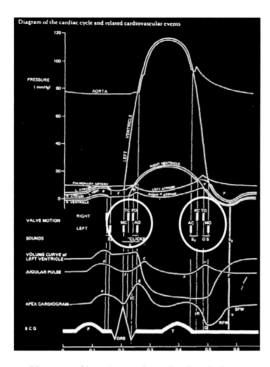

Diagram of heart sounds and valve timing

The pulmonic valve is located in the superoanterior region of the right ventricle. The normal valve has three cusps, the anterior, right, and left. Adjacent to each cusp lies the pulmonary artery wall that forms the pulmonic valve sinuses of Valsalva. The pulmonic trunk is posterior to the right ventricle and bifurcates into the right and left pulmonary artery. The pulmonic valve is normally opened during systole and closed during diastole carrying mostly deoxygenated blood to the lungs.

Pulmonic stenosis in adults is usually a result of congenital disease. It may occur along with other lesions, but most commonly Tetralogy of Fallot. Signs and symptoms of pulmonic stenosis may include cyanosis, exertional dyspnea, jugular venous distension, and a systolic ejection murmur.

The most common form of right ventricular outflow tract obstruction is pulmonic valve stenosis. The pulmonic cusps are thickened and domed with an abnormally small orifice. There may be

post-stenotic dilatation of the pulmonary artery. Since right ventricular outflow tract flow is restricted, right atrial enlargement may occur and a right to left shunt develops through the foramen ovale. When pulmonic stenosis is critical, cyanosis results due to the diminished pulmonary venous return and the desaturation of blood caused by the right to left atrial shunt.

The pulmonic valve is best visualized in a parasternal short axis view at the aortic valve and right ventricular outflow tract level. Doppler findings with pulmonic stenosis are similar to those with aortic stenosis. Flow distal to the site of stenosis will be high velocity and turbulent. The same calculations used for aortic stenosis can be applied to pulmonic stenosis. The pulmonic valve peak and mean velocities and pressure gradients and valve area should be quantified.

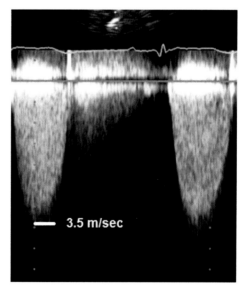

Pulmonic Stenosis

115

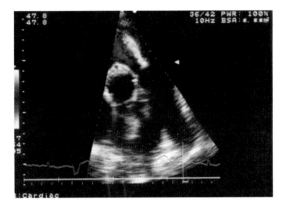

CFI Pulmonic Regurgitation

The 2-D exam of the valve may demonstrate the valve doming in diastole, increased pulmonary artery size, asymmetrical septal hypertrophy, and right ventricular hypertrophy. The right ventricle may range from small to normal in size.

Pulmonary atresia, or an absence of the valve may occur. Pulmonary atresia is commonly identified by the lack of valve motion. The interventricular septum may be intact leaving the interatrial septum as the only flow connection to the right heart. The valve region may have a fibrous membrane, the pulmonary trunk may be funnel shaped, hypoplastic, or slightly larger than normal. Often, right ventricular hypertrophy and a small right ventricle is noted. A small right ventricle is suggestive of either tricuspid atresia, pulmonary atresia with intact ventricular septum or pulmonary atresia with ventricular septal defect.

The distal portion of the pulmonary artery may have a blood supply as a result of a patent ductus arteriosus. **Patent ductus arteriosus** can be difficult to identify on the echocardiogram, especially in the adult. Pulmonary atresia also occurs in patients with transposition of the great arteries, Tetralogy of Fallot, and ventricular septal defects.

The echocardiogram demonstrates two types of echo patterns commonly seen with pulmonary atresia. One results in a short distance between the right ventricular outflow tract and main pulmonary artery with a membrane between them. In the other case, the proximal outflow tract is tapered. The pulmonary outflow tract starts some distance distally and increases gradually in diameter as it nears the pulmonary artery bifurcation. If there is no ventricular septal defect, then the right ventricle is usually small and an atrial shunt right to left is present.

The most common form of cyanotic heart disease is **Tetralogy of Fallot**. This disease is characterized by the following:

- A large anterior malalignment interventricular septal defect.
- A large overriding aorta. The aorta overrides the defect.
- A small pulmonary artery with stenosis. The stenosis can vary in location.
- Probable right ventricular hypertrophy.

There are variations of Tetralogy of Fallot, but the two main characteristics that need to exist are the ventricular septal defect and pulmonic stenosis. In some cases of Tetralogy of Fallot, the ventricular septal defect is large, but the pulmonary stenosis is mild to moderate. The patient may be acyanotic or may be referred to as having "pink" Tetralogy of Fallot. Shunts may be bi-directional or left to right. If there is severe pulmonic stenosis, the patient is cyanotic, and the shunt is usually right to left. Pulmonic stenosis may occur in four different locations or variations of these locations. Pulmonic stenosis can occur at the site of the infundibulum, pulmonary valve, subinfundibular, or the pulmonary trunk. The subinfundibular region is the least likely location while the infundibulum and

116

pulmonary valve regions are the most common sites.

Other congenital cardiac anomalies that may be associated with pulmonic stenosis are: persistent left superior vena cava, right aortic arch, abnormalities of the pulmonary artery and branches, absent pulmonary valve, incompetent aortic valve, and coronary artery anatomy variation.

The 2-D exam of Tetralogy of Fallot utilizes the parasternal long axis view to identifying the ventricular septal defect and an overriding, enlarged aorta. Right ventricular hypertrophy may be present.

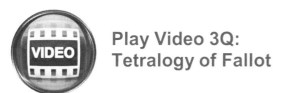

Play Video 3Q: Tetralogy of Fallot

The M-mode indications of pulmonic stenosis are an increased A wave, greater than 7mm, and an increased right ventricular ejection time.

The continuous wave Doppler determines the peak pressure gradient of the ventricular septal defect. Color flow imaging is most helpful in locating shunt flow in the parasternal long and short axis, apical, and subcostal views. Pulmonic stenosis can also be assessed using the modified Bernoulli equation. The flow typically is obtained in a high parasternal short axis view at the level of the aortic valve, right ventricular outflow tract, and pulmonary artery. Pulmonic, tricuspid, and aortic regurgitation may also be present.

A less common etiology for pulmonic stenosis is **carcinoid syndrome**. As discussed with tricuspid stenosis, the disease is a result of malignant carcinoid tumors and usually occurs in

the heart after hepatic metastasis. Approximately one-half of patients with carcinoid heart syndrome have right heart involvement. If the pulmonic valve is affected, a pearly white, fibrous scarring causes the stenosis and retraction of the valve.

Pulmonary Regurgitation

Pulmonic regurgitation or insufficiency is leakage of blood back into the right ventricular outflow tract. This may occur during part or all of diastole depending on the severity. As with the tricuspid valve, there is a small amount of regurgitation that is considered normal or physiologic in most patients.

Clinically, patients with pulmonic regurgitation may have a diastolic murmur that is very difficult to hear. They may have symptoms of shortness of breath. Pulmonary regurgitation may be the result of pulmonic stenosis, carcinoid syndrome, pulmonary hypertension, vegetations, post-operative valvotomy, and more rarely, myxomatous valve disease.

The 2-D exam on patients with pulmonic regurgitation may demonstrate enlargement of the right ventricular outflow tract and right ventricle, paradoxical septal motion when a right ventricular volume overload is present, enlargement of the pulmonary artery, and right atrial enlargement.

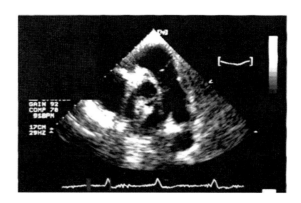

Dilated Pulmonary Artery and Bifurcation

117

The M-mode exam may show an enlarged right ventricle with paradoxical septal motion resulting from the right ventricular volume overload. Rarely, diastolic fluttering of the tricuspid leaflet may be noted. If pulmonary hypertension is present, the pulmonic valve may have the "Flying W" sign or mid systolic notching.

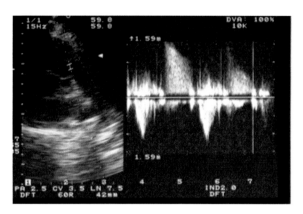

Pulmonic Regurgitation

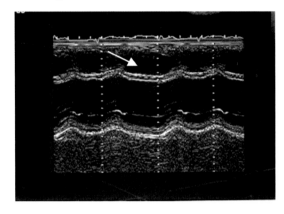

Paradoxical Septal Motion

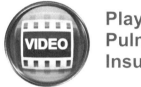

Play Video 3R.
Pulmonic
Insufficiency

The color flow imaging exam of pulmonary regurgitation displays the regurgitation as red or shades of red in the right ventricular outflow tract. The length, width, and height of the jet helps to determine the severity. The pulsed Doppler exam will demonstrate regurgitant flow displayed above the zero baseline. The intensity and shape of the continuous wave Doppler signal may indicate severe regurgitation. Holodiastolic flow reversal may be seen in the pulmonary artery if significant regurgitation is present. A pulmonary artery end diastolic pressure can be obtained by Bernoulli on the pulmonary regurgitation end diastolic velocity plus the right atrial pressure.

Endocarditis

Endocarditis is defined as an inflammation of the lining membrane of the heart. Typically, endocarditis involves the valves rather than the chambers, but either or both may be affected. Endocarditis may also occur at the site of AV fistulas, septal defects, and patent ductus arteriosus. Endocarditis or vegetations of the heart usually occur on already damaged valves. The following conditions render the heart susceptible to endocarditis:

- Previous valvulitis such as rheumatic valve disease or some other form of valve damage.
- Congenital heart lesions such as ventricular septal defects, patent ductus arteriosus, and bicuspid valve.
- Previous heart surgery such as valve replacement or repair and in-dwelling catheters.
- Patients who are immuno-suppressed, such as long term use of steroids.
- Patients who are IV drug users.

118

- Patients with a portal of entry such as dental work.

Endocarditis is classified into four groups: **rheumatic, infective, non-bacterial thrombotic, and atypical verrucous.**

Infective endocarditis (usually bacterial in origin) commonly is the result of enterococci or streptococcus viridans. Clinically, patient's present with a fever of unknown origin, positive blood cultures, and often a new murmur that may change. Patients may have embolic events. In acute bacterial endocarditis, Janeway lesions may be found. Janeway lesions are small, painless, red-blue macular lesions located on the patient's palms and soles of their feet. Osler nodes are also a possible finding with acute bacterial endocarditis. Osler nodes are small, raised, red, tender areas on the finger and toe pads caused by infected emboli from the heart. Splinter hemorrhages and hematuria may also be present.

Infective endocarditis can be classified into two types, acute and subacute. Acute is a rapid onset and is usually called by Staphylococcus aureus. Subacute bacterial endocarditis occurs from organisms of low grade virulence. These organisms invade areas already damaged by previous heart disease. Bacterial endocarditis usually affects left sided heart valves first. The aortic valve is the most common valve affected.

Rheumatic endocarditis is less prevalent, occurring after a bout of rheumatic fever.

Non-bacterial thrombotic endocarditis is often found in patients with malignancies or lupus. It is similar to infective endocarditis, however the vegetations are usually small and located at the base of the leaflets. Clinical and bacteriology information is necessary for the diagnosis.

Atypical verrucous is a non-bacterial form of endocarditis that is a result of an accumulation of debris in the endocardium. This is usually associated with wasting diseases such as lupus. Transthoracic echocardiography is fairly sensitive for the detection of endocarditis. Approximately 60-80 % of the time the 2-D exam will show irregular, echogenic areas or masses located on the valve surfaces. Vegetations as a rule do not usually restrict valve motion and may actually cause the valve to prolapse or become flail.

Aortic and pulmonic vegetations tend to occur on the ventricular sides of the valves, but may become large enough to extend around the other side or involve the chambers. **Mitral and tricuspid vegetations** usually occur on the atrial sides of the valves. Ultrasound may not detect vegetations that are less than 3mm in size. In some cases, more than one valve may have vegetations.

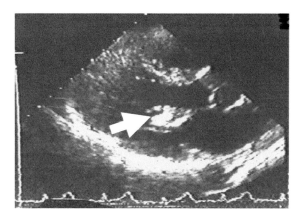

PLAX view of mitral valve vegetations seen on the atrial side of the anterior valve leaflet

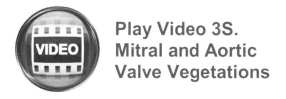

Play Video 3S.
Mitral and Aortic
Valve Vegetations

The M-mode appearance of vegetations is less diagnostic. Usually a thickening of the leaflets on the affected valve will be seen and valve motion is usually unrestricted.

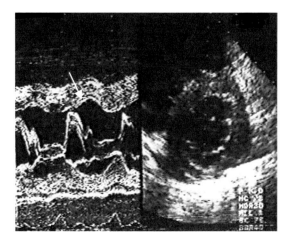

M-mode Mitral Valve Endocarditis

False positive appearances of valve vegetations may be due to Lambl's excrescence on the aortic valve. This appears as a linear echo on the ventricular side of the leaflet. Lambl's excrescence is a small fibroelastic protrusion seen in older patients. Calcifications of the Arantius nodules may also confuse the diagnosis of vegetations. The Arantius nodules are located at the aortic cusp tips and may become calcified with age. Beam width artifacts may cause the appearance of vegetations. Prosthetic valves often have thickened, calcified areas that may either appear as a vegetation or obscure a vegetation. Prosthetic valve thrombus may be mistaken for a vegetation. Transesophageal ultrasound has proven invaluable for the detection of vegetations, especially on patients with prosthetic valves.

Tricuspid valve vegetations may be viewed from a parasternal inflow view, short axis, or apical view. Tricuspid vegetations occur most often in patients who are IV drug abusers. These patients typically have large vegetations caused by the staphylococcus aureus infection. A frequent complication of tricuspid vegetations are septic pulmonary emboli.

The least common site for a valvular vegetation is the pulmonic valve. If a pulmonic valve vegetation occurs, endocarditis is already present on one or more other valves. The pulmonic valve vegetation is also usually seen on patients who are IV drug abusers or patients with right-sided catheters. There is a high mortality rate with pulmonic vegetations and surgical intervention may be indicated.

The Doppler findings with endocarditis are usually those of valvular dysfunction such as regurgitation, perforation, and possibly fistula tracts. Regurgitant jets as a result of vegetations are often eccentric and may be multiple. When long standing valve disease is present, left ventricular systolic dysfunction may be noted. Pulmonary artery pressures may be elevated in patients with mitral regurgitation that may result in elevated left atrial pressures. Aortic regurgitation may cause high end-diastolic ventricular pressures.

PROSTHETIC VALVES

Prosthetic valves fall into three basic types: homograft's, tissue valves or bioprosthesis, and mechanical valves.

Homograft's are human aortic valves that are harvested and cryopreserved. Usually the aortic valve, ascending aorta, and anterior leaflet are saved and trimmed at the time of surgery. These homograft's are usually used for pulmonic and aortic valve replacements.

Homograft's do not usually make good atrioventricular valve replacements since a supporting prosthetic structure is usually needed. Valve orifices tend to be slightly smaller than the normal native valves so velocities are slightly higher. **Bioprosthetic valves** are tissue valves. They are made of three biologic leaflets that are structured similar to the aortic valve. The valve leaflets are heterograft's of porcine or pig valves origin, but bovine or cow pericardium may be used and constructed to function like human leaflets. The heterograft is placed on a cloth covered metal support that functions as the aortic annulus with a raised stent located at each of the commissures. The variations in the support and types of leaflets account for the different names of each bioprosthetic valve available commercially.

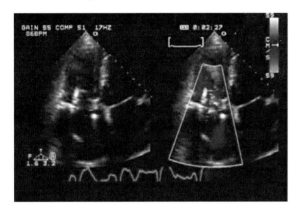

Normal Bioprosthetic Tricuspid Valve

Carpenter-Edwards valves may be porcine or pericardial valves. There are Hancock porcine valves, Ionescu-Shiley bovine pericardial valves and so on. All of these tissue valves are similar in the fact that they are tri-leaflet and have a circular orifice. They have flow patterns like native valves which are laminar with a blunt flow profile.

Tissue valves usually have a normally smaller valve area than native valves resulting in a normally high velocity flow through the valve. The support structures of tissue valves may limit the acoustic properties of the ultrasound. It is not unusual to see small amounts of regurgitation with prosthetic valves. If the bioprosthetic valve is a mitral valve the inflow is directed differently than in a native mitral valve. A bioprosthetic mitral valve has the flow to the left ventricle directed anteriorly and medial towards the interventricular septum rather than the apex. This causes a reversed vortex effect in mid diastole.

There are three basic types of **Mechanical valves**, however there are several variations of these available commercially. The **ball-cage valves** have a metal cage that has a spherical occluder contained within. It functions somewhat like a snorkel. The blood flows in this valve when it is in the open position across the sewing ring, around the ball occluder, and around all the struts. A small amount of regurgitation will be seen around the ball when it closes. An example of this type of valve is the Starr-Edwards valve.

The **tilting-disc valve** has a single circular disc that opens at an angle to the annulus. The disc is constrained by a central strut. The flow through this valve is through two openings one that is larger than the other. Flow is asymmetrical along the surface. Examples are Omniscience and Bjork-Shiley valves. The floating disk valve or Beall is no longer used.

The third type of mechanical valve is the **bi-leaflet valve.** This has two, hemicircular disks, that are hinged open. These form two large lateral openings and one small central opening. The St. Jude's valve is an example of a bileaflet valve. Flow through this valve is more complex. When the leaflets are open there are two, large lateral orifices and a small, central slit-like orifice. This type of valve shows velocity profiles of three peaks with high velocities in the orifice center. The localized pressure/ gradients of this type of valve's flow is often much higher than the overall pressure gradient.

The causes of prosthetic valve dysfunction can be much different from causes of native valve dysfunction. Tissue degeneration is one cause of a bioprosthetic valve to dysfunction. This is usually a process of slow, increasing degeneration. The leaflets become fibrocalcific resulting in stenosis and or regurgitation. When the leaflet in these valves tear, the patient usually presents with a sudden onset of a honking noise in the chest and acute heart failure.

Mechanical valves may fail due to poor design or wear and tear. Stenosis of a mechanical valve is often due to thrombus or pannus ingrowth. Pannus ingrowth is superficial vascular tissue that forms over an area of irritation. Other complications of prosthetic valves include greater than normal amounts of regurgitation usually due to a loss of sutures around the sewing ring and perivalvular leaks. Regurgitation may also be a result of endocarditis.

Valvuloplasty may be done to repair rather than replace valves. Tricuspid valvuloplasty is performed more often than tricuspid valve replacement. Tricuspid valvuloplasty is usually done in conjunction with a mitral valve replacement to control tricuspid regurgitation. This procedure may be referred to as a De Vega annuloplasty. Carpenter rings are usually used in the mitral valve as a support to the valve.

The following is a review of normal findings in prosthetic valves:

- A high percentage of prosthetic valves have a small amount of normal regurgitation.
- Normal flow velocities are usually higher in prosthetic valves.
- Prosthetic mitral valves usually have lower velocities than aortic valves due to their larger size.

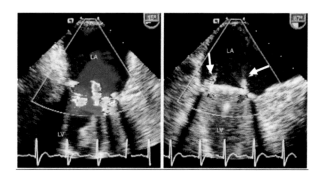

Normal bileaflet prosthetic valve
with some regurgitation

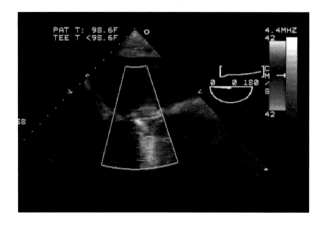

Normal CFI of St. Jude's prosthetic
valve with higher central velocity

Normal AVR Hemodynamics

	Peak Velocity	Mean Gradient
Heterograft	2.4	13.3
Ball-cage	3.2	23.0
Bjork-Shiley	2.5	13.9
St. Jude	2.5	14.4
Homograft	1.9	7.7
Medtronic-Hall	2.4	13.6

Normal MVR Hemodynamics

	Peak Velocity	Mean Gradient
Heterograft	1.6	4.1
Ball-cage	1.8	4.9
Bjork-Shiley	1.7	4.1
St. Jude	1.6	4.0

The 2-D examination of the prosthetic valve may be limited due to reverberation artifacts and dense acoustic shadows. 2-D examination may demonstrate some valve motion, the size of the cardiac chambers, and the motion and thickness of the walls.

M-mode findings are limited to the size of the chambers and wall thickness.

The Doppler exam is the most accurate method to evaluate the valves. Remember: a small degree of regurgitation is common. Stenosis of the valves can be determined by the use of pressure gradients and by calculating valve areas.

When evaluating a patient with a prosthetic valve the following information should be obtained:

- Peak and mean valve velocity.
- This needs to be compared to the type and size of valve.
- Peak and mean pressure gradients.
- Evaluation of regurgitation and the degree of regurgitation.
- Chamber size and wall thickness
- Systolic function
- Estimate pulmonary artery pressure if possible.

The following are echocardiographic indications of prosthetic valve dysfunction:

- Decreased valve area as calculated by continuity equation or pressure half time.
- Increasing flow velocity across the valve.
- Increasing amounts of regurgitation.
- Increasing intensity of continuous wave Doppler signals of regurgitant flow.
- Recurring pulmonary hypertension.
- Left ventricular hypertrophy.
- "Rocking" valve with perivalvular leak.

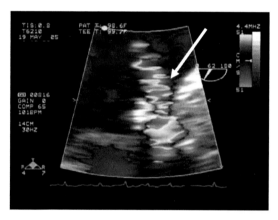

Perivalvular Leak

VALVULAR HEART DISEASE QUIZ

1. The most common cause of mitral stenosis is:
   a. myxomatous degeneration
   b. cleft mitral valve
   c. syphilis
   d. rheumatic fever

2. A commonly seen arrhythmia with mitral stenosis is:
   a. atrial fibrillation
   b. sinus tachycardia
   c. premature ventricular contractions
   d. premature atrial contraction

3. Name the type of mitral valve deformity that occurs when both chordae insert into a single papillary muscle.
   a. cleft mitral valve
   b. parachute mitral valve
   c. Ebstein's anomaly
   d. mitral valve prolapse

4. Which of the following is not a probable cause for calcification of the mitral valve annulus?
   a. metabolic disease
   b. aging
   c. hypertension
   d. tricuspid regurgitation

5. The most common tumor mass to cause mitral valve obstruction is:
   a. rhabdomyoma
   b. sarcoma
   c. myxoma
   d. teratoma

6. Which of the following is NOT a probable finding on the M-mode exam of a patient with mitral stenosis?
   a. flying W" sign of Pulmonic valve
   b. flattened E-F slope
   c. systolic anterior motion ALMV
   d. reduced D-E distance

7. When the mitral leaflets are fused together the 2-D appearance may be termed:
   a. "candle flame"
   b. "hockey stick"
   c. "flying W"
   d. "b-bump"

8. Severe mitral stenosis is considered when the mitral valve area is:
   a. < 10 cm²
   b. < 1.0 cm²
   c. < 2.0 cm²
   d. < 15 cm²

9. Severe mitral stenosis is considered when the mean pressure gradient is:
   a. 2-4 mmHg
   b. > 5 mmHg
   c. > 10 mmHg
   d. > 8 mmHg

10. Barlow's syndrome is another term used when referring to:
    a. parachute mitral valve
    b. mitral valve prolapse
    c. cleft mitral valve
    d. myxomatous mitral valve

11. On the M-mode tracing of the mitral valve, a prolapse is considered when the leaflet(s) are displaced _____ below the C-D points?
    a. 3-5 cm
    b. 1-2 cm
    c. > 3 mm
    d. > 3 cm

12. Which leaflet of the mitral valve is more commonly involved in a spontaneous rupture of the chordae tendineae?
    a. posterior leaflet
    b. anterior leaflet
    c. affects both the same
    d. septal leaflet

13. When one of the mitral valve leaflets are flail, the leaflet tip points toward the:
    a. left ventricle
    b. left atrium
    c. aortic valve
    d. does not change position

14. This M-mode tracing of the mitral valve is primarily suggestive of:

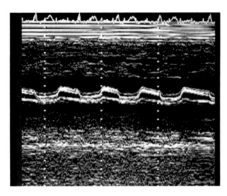

   a. mitral stenosis
   b. mitral regurgitation
   c. mitral valve prolapse
   d. flail mitral valve

15. The most common cause of papillary muscle dysfunction is:
   a. cardiomyopathy
   b. defective muscular development
   c. endomyocardial disease
   d. coronary artery disease

16. This 2-D picture of the mitral valve suggests:

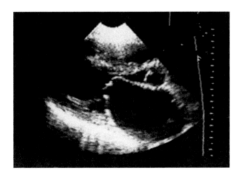

   a. mitral stenosis
   b. mitral valve prolapse
   c. mitral annulus calcification
   d. mitral regurgitation

17. When the mitral leaflet is flail left ventricular function is commonly:
   a. hypokinetic
   b. hyperkinetic
   c. akinetic
   d. normal

18. What flow velocity can be used to calculate pulmonary artery pressure?
   a. mitral regurgitation
   b. aortic regurgitation
   c. pulmonic stenosis
   d. tricuspid regurgitation

19. On the Doppler exam, severe mitral valve regurgitation is indicated when:
   a. MV prolapse > 3 mm
   b. systolic reversal of pulmonary vein flow is detected
   c. peak systolic velocity > 4m/s
   d. regurgitant jet is eccentric

20. Severe aortic stenosis is considered when the aortic valve area is:
   a. > 2 cm²
   b. < 2 cm²
   c. < 1 cm²
   d. < 1.5 cm²

21. To calculate the peak pressure gradient in aortic stenosis, what equation is used?
   a. modified Bernoulli equation
   b. modified Simpson's equation
   c. continuity equation
   d. pressure half-time

22. When severe aortic stenosis is present, the left ventricle walls usually:
   a. thin
   b. hypertrophy
   c. stay normal
   d. become decreased in echogenicity

23. The most common congenital malformation of the heart is:
    a. unicuspid aortic valve
    b. parachute aortic valve
    c. cleft aortic valve
    d. bicuspid aortic valve

24. Another possible coexisting defect seen with bicuspid aortic valve is:
    a. cleft tricuspid valve
    b. coarctation of the aorta
    c. parachute mitral valve
    d. cleft mitral valve

25. In severe cases of aortic stenosis the aortic root may:
    a. decrease in size
    b. dilate
    c. hypertrophy
    d. decrease in echogenicity

26. Severe aortic stenosis is considered when the mean pressure gradient is:
    a. > 50 mmHg
    b. > 40 mmHg
    c. > 30 mmHg
    d. > 20 mmHg

27. Type I bicuspid aortic valve has the coronary arteries arising:
    a. anterior to the anterior cusp
    b. posterior to the posterior cusp
    c. anterior and posterior to each respective cusp
    d. to the right and left of the respective cusp

28. When the aortic valve is bicuspid, a larger cusp may be the result of a:
    a. raphe
    b. cleft
    c. calcification
    d. parachute deformity

29. Which of the following is NOT a cause of aortic root dilatation? a. mitral stenosis
    b. Marfan's syndrome
    c. hypertension
    d. cystic medial necrosis

30. The "water balloon" appearance is associated with:
    a. bicuspid aortic valve
    b. unicuspid valve
    c. Marfan's syndrome
    d. cystic medial necrosis

31. The most common risk factor for aortic dissection is:
    a. trauma
    b. chronic hypertension
    c. atherosclerosis
    d. bicuspid valve

32. Fine fluttering of the anterior mitral leaflet may suggest:
    a. mitral regurgitation
    b. aortic stenosis
    c. aortic regurgitation
    d. mitral stenosis

33. When chronic aortic regurgitation is present, the left ventricle shape may become:
    a. conical
    b. spherical
    c. elliptical
    d. octagonal

34. This CW Doppler tracing of the aortic valve suggests:

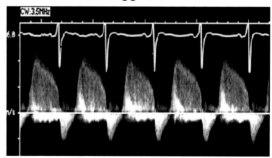

    a. aortic regurgitation
    b. aortic stenosis
    c. bicuspid valve
    d. Marfan's syndrome

35. Severe aortic regurgitation is 100% sensitive when:
    a. holodiastolic flow reversal is in the descending aorta
    b. holodiastolic flow reversal is in the ascending aorta
    c. pressure half-time of the aortic regurgitation is > 250 ms
    d. regurgitation spectral tracing is box-like in appearance

36. If the cause of tricuspid stenosis is rheumatic valvulitis, what other lesion almost always coexists?
    a. aortic stenosis
    b. pulmonic stenosis
    c. mitral stenosis
    d. aortic regurgitation

37. An auscultatory finding in tricuspid stenosis of an increased intensity of the diastolic murmur with inspiration is referred to as:
    a. DeRosier's sign
    b. Carvallo's sign
    c. Murphy's sign
    d. Epstein's sign

38. Severe tricuspid stenosis is considered when the tricuspid valve area is:
    a. < 3 cm²
    b. < 2 cm²
    c. < 1.5 cm²
    d. < 4 cm²

39. Tricuspid stenosis resulting from a metastatic tumor is referred to as:
    a. endomyocardial stenosis
    b. carcinoid syndrome
    c. fibroelastosis
    d. tricuspid atresia

40. Up to 10% of all cardiac disease is a result of endomyocardial fibrosis in:
    a. South America
    b. United States
    c. Africa
    d. Central America

41. Which tricuspid leaflet is almost always involved in Ebstein's anomaly?
    a. septal
    b. anterior
    c. posterior
    d. all are usually affected equally

42. Ebstein's anomaly is considered when the separation of the tricuspid valve from the mitral valve is:
    a. > 5 mm
    b. > 3 cm
    c. > 2 cm
    d. > 10 mm

43. When severe tricuspid regurgitation is suspected, systolic flow reversal may be noted in the:
    a. IVC
    b. SVC
    c. middle hepatic vein
    d. none of the above
    e. all of the above

44. A normal right ventricular systolic pressure is:
    a. < 35-40 mmHg
    b. < 45-50 mmHg
    c. < 55-60 mmHg
    d. < 65-70 mmHg

45. Pulmonic stenosis in adults is usually the result of:
    a. carcinoid disease
    b. pulmonic atresia
    c. congenital disease
    d. fibroelastosis

46. The best view to evaluate the pulmonic valve is the:
    a. apical
    b. parasternal long axis
    c. parasternal short axis
    d. suprasternal

47. The least likely region for pulmonic stenosis to occur in patients with Tetralogy of Fallot is the:
   a. infundibulum
   b. pulmonic valve
   c. pulmonic trunk
   d. subinfundibular

48. Infective endocarditis is usually the result of:
   a. virus
   b. bacteria
   c. lupus
   d. malignancy

49. A non-bacterial form of endocarditis that results in an accumulation of debris in the endocardium is:
   a. non-bacterial thrombotic
   b. rheumatic
   c. atypical verrucous
   d. infective

50. Ultrasound may not detect vegetations that are:
   a. < 6 mm
   b. < 3 cm
   c. < 1 cm
   d. < 3 mm

51. A small fibroelastic protrusion seen on the aortic valve in older patients may represent:
   a. Osler nodes
   b. Janeway lesions
   c. Lambl's excrescence
   d. Chiari's network

52. Tricuspid valve vegetations occur most often in patients with:
   a. lupus
   b. I.V. drug abuse
   c. Epstein's anomaly
   d. tricuspid atresia

53. A frequent complication of tricuspid valve vegetation is:
   a. left ventricular thrombus
   b. left atrial thrombus
   c. septic pulmonary emboli
   d. right ventricular hypertrophy

54. The least common site for endocarditis is:
   a. aortic valve
   b. mitral valve
   c. tricuspid valve
   d. pulmonic valve

55. Which one of the following prosthetic valve types is made from human aortic valves?
   a. bioprosthesis
   b. homograft's
   c. heterograft's
   d. none of the above

56. The most common cause of a bio-prosthetic valve to dysfunction is:
   a. bad design
   b. pannus ingrowth
   c. tissue degeneration
   d. endocarditis

57. Which of the following is NOT a cause of mechanical valve failure?
   a. pannus ingrowth
   b. valve leaflet tears
   c. bad design
   d. loss of sutures around the sewing ring

58. When a tricuspid valve repair is done in conjunction with a mitral valve replacement it may be called a _____ annuloplasty.
   a. Janeway
   b. DeVega
   c. DeRosier
   d. Beall

59. What is the abnormality indicated on the image below?

    a. mitral stenosis
    b. mitral valve endocarditis
    c. mitral valve annular calcification
    d. parachute deformity of the mitral valve

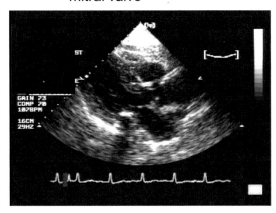

60. The apical four chamber view on the image below may be an indication of all of the following EXCEPT:
    a. atrial septal defect
    b. severe tricuspid regurgitation
    c. pulmonary hypertension
    d. aortic stenosis

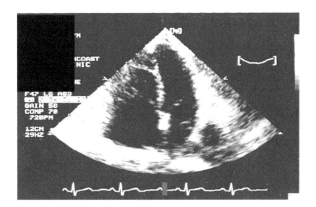

61. Which disease state can cause the mitral valve pressure half-time to be incorrect?
    a. aortic stenosis
    b. aortic insufficiency
    c. mitral valve prolapse
    d. pulmonic regurgitation

62. What may cause the following abnormality seen on the CF image below?
    a. VSD
    b. Papillary muscle dysfunction
    c. Coronary artery disease
    d. Bicuspid aortic valve

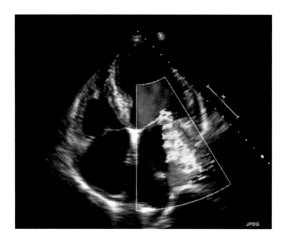

63. From what view is the following Doppler of Aortic stenosis taken?
    a. Apex
    b. Apical 5 chamber view
    c. Right parasternal
    d. None of the above

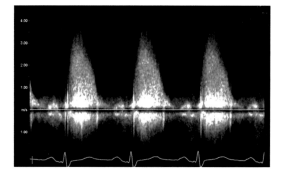

64. Diagnose the following M-mode?
    a. Systolic anterior motion
    b. Fine fluttering of the MV
    c. Mitral valve prolapse
    d. Mitral stenosis

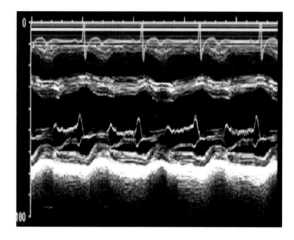

65. What is the most likely cause for the following Apical 4C image?
    a. Mitral valve prolapse
    b. Aortic stenosis
    c. Coronary artery disease
    d. Carcinoid heart disease

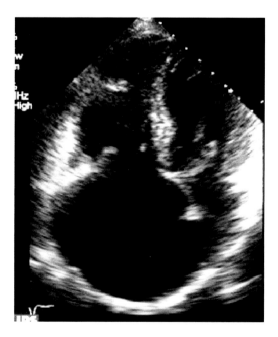

66. Indicate at what point you would measure the diameter of the IVC on the image below?
    a.
    b.
    c.
    d.

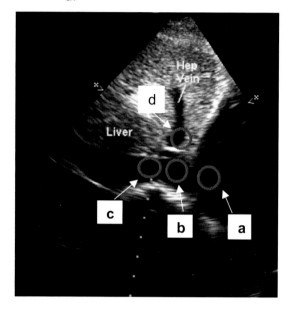

67. Diagnose the following image?
    a. pulmonic regurgitation
    b. mitral regurgitation
    c. tricuspid regurgitation
    d. aortic regurgitation

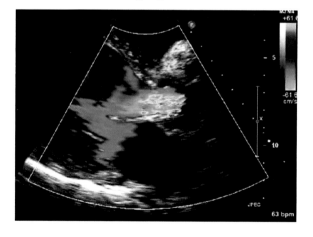

68. Diagnose the following M-mode of the LV?

    a. Mitral valve prolapse
    b. Septal hypokinesis
    c. Left ventricular hypertrophy
    d. Left ventricular dilatation

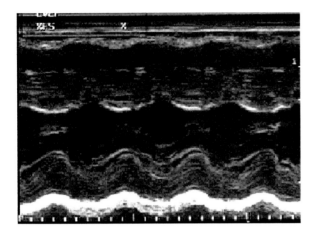

69. What is the AVA with the given information?

LVOT Diameter	2.1 cm
LVOT Velocity	1.0 m/sec
Aortic Velocity	4.2 m/sec
Aortic Mean Vel.	3.5 m/sec

    a. 2.46 cm^2
    b. $.59 \text{ cm}^2$
    c. $.82 \text{ cm}^2$
    d. 2.0 cm^2

70. Determine the RVSP with the given information"

TR velocity 3.4 m/sec with normal IVC

    a. 51 mmHg
    b. 46 mmHg
    c. 31 mmHg
    d. 26 mmHg

71. Acute mitral regurgitation typically causes the LV to become:
    a. hypokinetic
    b. hyperkinetic
    c. akinetic
    d. none of the above

72. Choose three criteria the would signify severe mitral regurgitation:

    a. < 1.5 m/sec peak MV velocity
    b. > 1.5 m/sec peak MV velocity
    c. < 4 cm² Regurgitant jet area
    d. >8 cm² Regurgitant jet area
    e. 20% RJA/LAA
    f. 40% RJA/LAA

73. What is the PAEDP with the given information:

    PREDV 1.2 m/sec
    RAP 5 mmHg

    a. 6.4 mmHg
    b. 11 mmHg
    c. 15.3 mmHg
    d. 22 mmHg

74. Diagnose the image of the PSAX at the LV:
    a. Dilated LV
    b. RV pressure overload
    c. Left ventricular hypertrophy
    d. Mitral stenosis

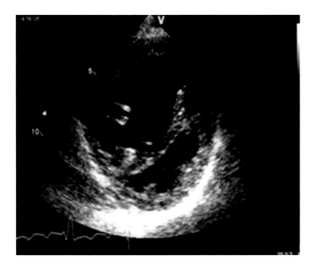

75. Select the 4 required pieces of information needed in order to perform a PISA calculation of mitral regurgitation:
    a. Aortic VTI
    b. Radius
    c. MV VTI
    d. MR peak velocity
    e. TV VTI
    f. MR VTI
    g. Aliasing velocity

76. What is the pressure gradient across Aortic valve for the given information:

    AoV Peak Velocity 4.2 m/sec

    a. 12 mmHg
    b. 18 mmHg
    c. 71 mmHg
    d. 81 mmHg

77. Diagnose the following M-mode:
    a. Mitral stenosis
    b. Left ventricular hypertrophy
    c. Mitral valve prolapse
    d. Systolic anterior motion

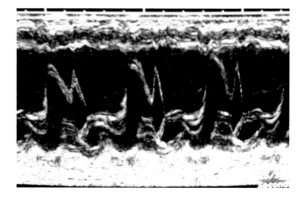

78. Diagnose the following image:
    a. Anterior motion of the posterior MV leaflet during diastole
    b. Systolic Anterior motion of the MV during diastole
    c. Posterior motion of the MV during systole
    d. Posterior motion of the anterior MV leaflet during diastole

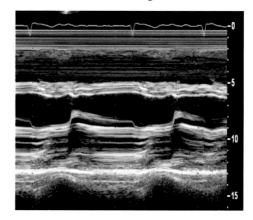

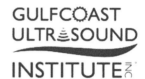

Section 4:

Pericardial Disease

Section 4: PERICARDIAL DISEASE

Objectives

Upon completion of this module you should be able to:

- Identify the echocardiographic findings associated with pericardial disease

- Recognize the etiologies of the various types of pericardial disease

- Differentiate pericardial and pleural fluid collections

- Apply quantitative measurements to applicable diseases

- Recognize the various types of pericardial diseases

Pericardial Disease

The heart is separated from the surrounding mediastinal structures by a double-walled, fibroserosal sac called the pericardium. The pericardium stops the heart from rotating excessively, prevents friction, and possible kinking of the great vessels. The epicardium or visceral pericardium adheres to the outer heart surface while the parietal pericardium adheres to the diaphragm, inner sternal surface, and adjacent pleural spaces. The visceral and parietal pericardium are continuous with each other. A space separating these layers contains approximately 5-10 ml of lubricating lymph fluid called the pericardial sac.

PERICARDITIS

When the pericardium becomes inflamed it is referred to as pericarditis. There are several etiologies for pericarditis. The etiologies for pericarditis are categorized into the following four groups: **Infections, malignancies, inflammatory, and intracardiac-pericardiac.**

Infections
- Post-viral (AIDS, echovirus, etc.)
- Bacterial infections
- Tuberculosis
- Others

Malignant
- Lymphoma
- Melanoma
- Direct extension of breast and lung cancer.
- Primary cardiac malignancies may be a cause, but are rare.

Inflammatory Processes
- Dressler's syndrome
- Uremia
- Collagen-vascular disease
- Post-op cardiac surgery

Intracardiac-Pericardial Communications
- Trauma
- Post catheter procedures such as valvuloplasty or atherectomy
- Left ventricular rupture after a myocardial infarction.

Pericarditis also results from unknown, or undetectable origins.

Typically, at some point in the disease patients with pericarditis develop a pericardial effusion, but it is not always detected or necessary to make the diagnosis.

Clinically, the patient usually has positional chest pain that is relieved by leaning forward, a pericardial rub with auscultation, and electrocardiographic changes. A pericardial rub or friction sound is a result of the rubbing of the roughened pericardial surfaces.

2-D and M-Mode findings of an effusion of varying size, or pericardial thickening may be seen, but the diagnosis of pericarditis is usually made clinically.

Constrictive pericarditis is a fibrous thickening, possibly with adherent calcifications, of the visceral and parietal layers of the pericardium. Constrictive pericarditis results in the impairment of diastolic ventricular filling caused by the surrounding rigid pericardium that acts somewhat like a box around the heart. Rapid, early diastolic filling stops abruptly due to the rising diastolic pressures, or in effect, the box is full.

Causes of Constrictive Pericarditis.
- Multiple episodes of pericarditis
- Radiation therapy
- Cardiac surgery
- Tuberculosis
- Coxsackie pericarditis
- Neoplasm
- Amyloidosis
- Trauma
- Foreign body
- Systemic lupus erythematosus
- Rheumatoid arthritis

Signs and symptoms of constrictive pericarditis tend to be less intense due to the gradual onset of the disease. Elevated ventricular, atrial, and pulmonary systemic venous pressures may be noted. Patients may present with dyspnea, orthopnea, fatigue, and malaise due to low cardiac output. Physical findings of engorgement of neck veins, pleural effusions, hepatomegaly, ascites, and peripheral edema may also occur. In a small number of cases pulsus paradoxus may result. A pericardial knock may be heard in early diastole.

2-D imaging may demonstrate the pericardial thickening and an increase in echogenicity, especially if calcifications are present. Other possible findings associated with constrictive pericarditis are flattening of the diastolic wall motion, left atrial enlargement, and dilatation of the inferior vena cava and hepatic veins. Dilatation of the inferior vena cava and hepatic veins is suggested when the inferior vena cava measures 2.1 cm or greater as it enters into the right atrium, and no size variation is noted in these vessels with respiration.

The M-mode findings include pericardial thickening, paradoxical septal motion, flattening of the mid-diastolic left ventricular posterior wall motion, a short E-F slope, premature opening of the pulmonic valve, and left atrial enlargement. Left ventricular size and systolic function should be normal until late in the disease process.

The Doppler findings with constrictive pericarditis include a prominent Y descent in the hepatic vein or vena cava flow, a prominent E velocity with an early, rapid diastolic deceleration slope of the left ventricle inflow, and the A velocity of the left ventricle inflow will be small or missing.

With patient inspiration, there may be a mean increase of 20% of the left ventricular isovolumetric relaxation time. The isovolumetric relaxation time can be measured from the aortic valve closure to the opening of the mitral click. There is a greater than 25% difference from normal patients' with respiratory variations in the right ventricle/left ventricle diastolic filling. The right ventricle filling increases with inspiration and left ventricle filling decreases with inspiration. There is a prominent A wave, and blunted systolic flow during the left atrial filling phase of the pulmonary venous flow.

PERICARDIAL EFFUSION

If a larger than normal amount of fluid develops in the pericardial space, it is referred to as a **pericardial effusion**. Indications of a pericardial effusion may include distant heart sounds, a low voltage EKG, and an enlarged cardiac silhouette on a chest X-ray (cardiomegaly). The classification of the pericardial effusion depends upon the amount of fluid located between the parietal and visceral pericardium.

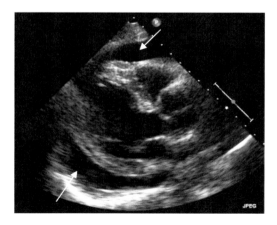

Parasternal Long Axis Small Anterior and Posterior Pericardial Effusion

Classification of Pericardial Effusion

Small	**< 0.5 cm**
Moderate	**0.5 to 2.0 cm**
Large	**> 2.0 cm**

*Source: TEXTBOOK of CLINICAL
ECHOCARDIOGRAPHY (Otto & Pearlman)*

A pericardial effusion appears as an echo-free space of varying size on the 2-D examination. If large enough, the effusion may be seen both posteriorly and anteriorly. In a large pericardial effusion, distant heart sounds producing a dullness in percussion is called Ewart's sign. In patients with pericardial effusions over a longer length of time, various fibrinous strands may be present and seen in the fluid. Infected or metastatic fluid may appear hazy. When an anterior only echo-free space is noted, a pericardial fat pad may be the cause rather than fluid.

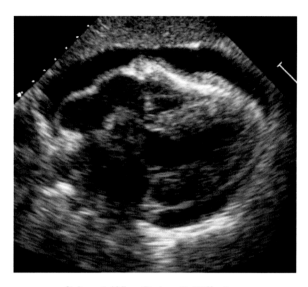

Subcostal View Pericardial Effusion

Effusions may be loculated or in pockets. This finding is more commonly seen with post-op patients, or patients with recurring pericardial disease, and may be a result of adhesions. If the fluid is loculated, or in a place that cannot be aspirated, even small effusions can cause hemodynamic problems. The parasternal, apical, and subcostal views best visualize pericardial effusions.

The M-mode tracing of a pericardial effusion demonstrates a flattening of the posterior pericardial reflection with an echo-free space and the moving epicardial reflection.

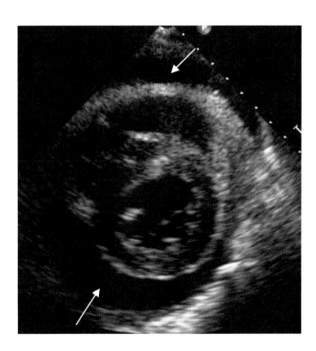

Short Axis Pericardial Effusion

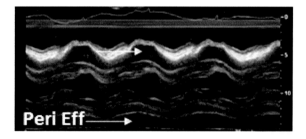

M-mode Small Pericardial Effusion

141

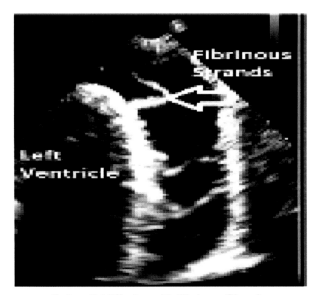

Pericardial Effusion with Fibrinous Strands

Cardiac tamponade results when the pressure in the pericardium is greater than the pressure in the cardiac chambers, resulting in impaired cardiac filling. When tamponade is complete, the diastolic pressures in all of the cardiac chambers are increased and equal to one another. The onset of pericardial tamponade depends on the rate and volume of the accumulation of fluid. Clinical indications of tamponade are tachycardia, hypotension, elevation of jugular venous pressures, and pulsus paradoxus. Pulsus paradoxus is a decline of greater than 10mmHg in systemic pressure with inspiration. Beck's triad describes three of the clinical indications which includes, increased venous pressure, decreased systolic blood pressure and muffled heart sounds.

The 2-D appearance of a large pericardial effusion typically demonstrates both anterior and posterior echo-free spaces, paradoxical motion of the interventricular septum and posterior wall, and a possible pseudo mitral valve prolapse. The M-mode has similar findings, as well as mid-systolic notching of the pulmonic valve, early closure of the aortic valve, and pseudo anterior motion of the mitral valve.

2-D Indications of Cardiac Tamponade

- Moderate to large pericardial effusion
- Right atrial systolic collapse that is greater than 1/3 of systole
- Reciprocal changes in volumes of right and left ventricle with respiration

If right atrial systolic collapse is present, it is 94% sensitive and 100% specific for the diagnosis of tamponade. Right ventricular diastolic collapse occurs as a result of intrapericardial pressures that exceed the right ventricular diastolic pressures. This finding can be seen when the right ventricular free wall is normal in thickness and compliance. The finding of right ventricle diastolic collapse is 60-90% sensitive in detecting tamponade, but 85-100% specific as compared to right atrial systolic collapse.

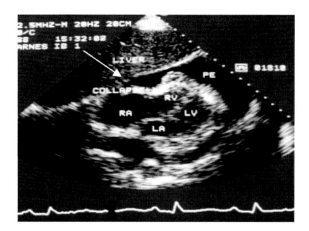

RV Diastolic Collapse with Tamponade

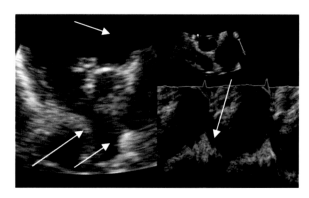

RA Systolic Collapse with Tamponade

142

Play Video 4A: PLAX Tamponade

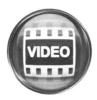

Play Video 4B: SAX/Apical Tamponade

DOPPLER INDICATIONS OF TAMPONADE

Marked decrease (>25%) in mitral valve velocity with inspiration; use 25 mm paper speed

Marked decrease (>25%) in aortic velocity with inspiration; use 25 mm paper speed

Marked respiratory variation of pulmonary veins

Inferior vena cava plethora.

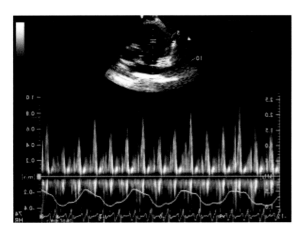

Greater than 25% decrease in MV Doppler seen in patients with cardiac tamponade

Inferior vena cava plethora is indicated when there is a less than 50% reduction in diameter of the inferior vena cava with inspiration. This observation should be made just before the inferior vena cava enters the right atrium. All of these echocardiographic findings may be helpful in the diagnosis of tamponade, but ultimately it is a clinical and hemodynamic diagnosis. There are also differing degrees of tamponade, therefore echocardiographic findings may vary. Usually when a pericardial effusion is not present, the diagnosis of tamponade can be excluded. Rarely, other mediastinal substrates may cause tamponade such as compression mass, or air due to barotrauma.

Differentiation of pericardial fluid from pleural fluid may be difficult. The parasternal long axis view can be extremely valuable for the differentiation of fluid collections around the heart. Typically, pericardial effusions stop at the level of the descending aorta, and may increase the distance between the heart and the descending aorta.

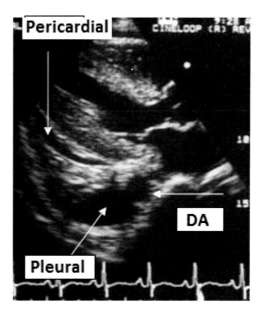

Pericardial and Pleural Effusions

Pleural effusions tend to extend beyond the descending aorta, and no separation should be noted between the descending aorta and the wall of the heart.

In instances of very large pericardial effusions, fluid may be seen around the left atrium in the oblique sinus. As suggested previously, an anterior only finding of fluid should be suspicious for fat rather than fluid. Do not confuse the coronary sinus or descending thoracic aorta for fluid. If anything, use these for landmarks for pleural versus pericardial fluid. Doppler or color flow imaging can help to define the descending aorta.

The apical views may be helpful in determining the extent of a pericardial effusion. Any fluid collection superior to the right atrium only, most likely represents a pleural rather than a pericardial effusion. Pleural effusions can also be detected by scanning the lateral aspect of the chest wall by the diaphragm/liver, or diaphragm/spleen interfaces.

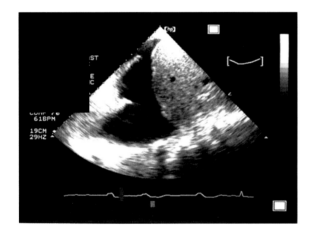

Large Right Pleural Effusion (Liver/Diaphragm Interface)

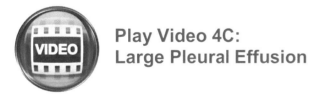

Play Video 4C:
Large Pleural Effusion

The subcostal view is helpful in locating pericardial effusion for echo- guided pericardiocentesis, however, the best site is the largest pocket of fluid that is located away from the diaphragm and lung.

Mistakes can be made when determining pericardial effusions. Echocardiography is considered the best technique to find pericardial fluid, but some conditions may be confusing. Fluid which has fibrous strands or clots may not look echo- free and may appear as surrounding tissue rather than fluid. Loculated collections, especially those located in difficult areas to view, may produce a false negative result.

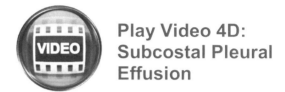

Play Video 4D:
Subcostal Pleural Effusion

If **pericardial cysts** or **pseudoaneurysms** are present, they can be confused for fluid collections. Remember, the patient's history is important in ruling in or out other possible cardiac conditions. Hiatal hernias may become quite large and be seen posterior to the heart resulting in a misdiagnosis of fluid or mass. Subphrenic abscesses may also occur. Large, dense mitral annular calcifications can cause an echo drop out that may look like fluid, especially on the M-mode exam.

PERICARDIAL TUMORS

Primary pericardial tumors are rare, however; approximately 75% of metastatic disease involves the pericardium and epicardium. Primary pericardial tumors include benign lipomas, fibromas, and hemangiomas. Malignant tumors are mesotheliomas or sarcomas

A rare finding in children are benign teratomas that grow in the pericardium becoming large and compressing other structures. Metastatic pericardial tumors are usually from the lung, breast, lymphoma, melanoma, and leukemia. Melanoma has the highest rate of metastasis to the pericardium, but is fairly uncommon. Lymphomas related to AIDS commonly have extensive cardiac involvement.

If pericardial fluid is noted on a patient with a known primary tumor, metastatic disease should be suspected. Fluid may have strands or thickening. Patients with malignancies and pericardial effusions may also develop radiation pericarditis associated with their therapy. Idiopathic pericarditis is a common finding in cancer patients. When a malignant pericardial effusion is detected, the prognosis is poor. The one-year survival rate is less than 50%.

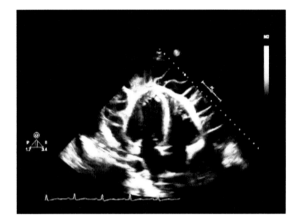

Malignant pericardial strands

PERICARDIAL DISEASE QUIZ

1. Which one of the following is NOT a category of pericarditis?
   a. infectious
   b. inflammatory
   c. intracardiac-pericardial communications
   d. atypical verrucous

2. Which of the following is NOT an inflammatory process associated with pericarditis?
   a. uremia
   b. Dressler's syndrome
   c. left ventricular rupture
   d. collagen-vascular disease

3. A friction sound caused by the rubbing of the roughened pericardial surfaces heard with auscultation is a:
   a. honking sound
   b. pericardial rub
   c. pericardial knock
   d. pericardial whine

4. Constrictive pericarditis results in impairment of:
   a. diastolic ventricular filling
   b. systolic ventricular emptying
   c. left atrial filling
   d. valve function

5. An auscultatory finding in constrictive pericarditis may be a:
   a. pericardial rub
   b. pericardial knock
   c. Carvallo's sign
   d. honking sound

6. Which of the following is NOT a 2-D finding associated with constrictive pericarditis?
   a. pericardial thickening
   b. increased diastolic wall motion
   c. flattening of the diastolic wall motion
   d. dilated IVC and hepatic veins

7. Which of the following is NOT a possible M-mode finding with constrictive pericarditis?
   a. paradoxical septal motion
   b. enlarged left ventricle
   c. short E-F slope
   d. flattening of the mid-diastolic posterior wall motion.

8. Fluid that stops at the level of the descending aorta and increases the distance between the heart and the descending aorta most likely represents a _____:
   a. pleural effusion
   b. pericardial effusion
   c. pericardial fat pad
   d. pericardial tumor

9. Loculated effusions are most often seen _____.
   a. with malignancy
   b. in post-op patients
   c. with pericarditis
   d. with tamponade

10. Which of the following is NOT a Doppler finding associated with constrictive pericarditis?
    a. small or missing A wave on the mitral valve inflow tracing
    b. prominent A wave on the left ventricle inflow tracing
    c. prominent Y descent in the IVC or hepatic vein flow
    d. prominent E wave on the left ventricular inflow.

11. A large pericardial effusion is considered when the separation between the parietal and visceral pericardium is:
    a. > 0.5 cm
    b. > 1.0 cm
    c. > 1.5 cm
    d. > 2.0 cm

12. When an anterior only echo-free space is noted on the 2-D exam a possible should be suspected.
    a. anterior effusion
    b. moderate effusion
    c. pericardial fat pad
    d. pleural effusion

13. This 2-D picture indicates:
    a. pericardial effusion
    b. pleural effusion
    c. both pericardial and pleural effusion
    d. prominent descending aorta

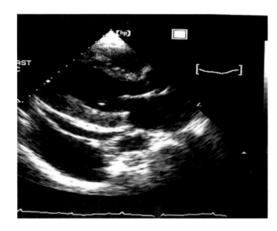

14. What finding on the 2-D exam is 100% specific for the diagnosis of cardiac tamponade?
    a. left ventricle diastolic collapse
    b. right atrial diastolic collapse lasting longer than 1/3 of diastole.
    c. right atrial systolic collapse lasting longer than 1/3 of systole
    d. right ventricular systolic collapse

15. A less than 50% reduction in diameter of the IVC with inspiration indicates:
    a. IVC integra
    b. IVC decompensation
    c. IVC decompression
    d. IVC plethora

16. Which view is helpful when performing pericardiocentesis:
    a. parasternal long axis
    b. parasternal short axis
    c. apical 4 chamber
    d. subcostal

17. The onset of pericardial tamponade depends on:
    a. rate of fluid accumulation
    b. volume of fluid accumulation
    c. location of fluid
    d. a & b
    e. b & c

18. A 25% decrease in the MV velocity with inspiration suggests:
    a. small pericardial effusion
    b. pericardial clot
    c. cardiac tamponade
    d. pericardial tumor

19. The PLA view on the image below suggests the finding of?
    a. right ventricular collapse
    b. right atrial collapse
    c. IVC plethora
    d. paradoxical septal motion

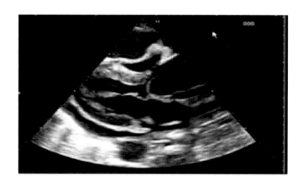

20. The M-mode tracing below indicates:
    a. pericardial effusion with pseudo prolapse
    b. pleural effusion
    c. pericardial and pleural effusions
    d. normal left ventricle

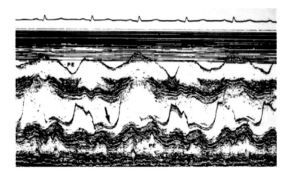

21. Which of the following is a malignant tumor:
    a. mesothelioma
    b. hemangioma
    c. lipoma
    d. fibroma

22. The image below was obtained from a right lateral position near the region of the diaphragm and indicates a:
    a. right pericardial effusion
    b. right pleural effusion
    c. tumor in the diaphragm
    d. normal diaphragm/liver interface

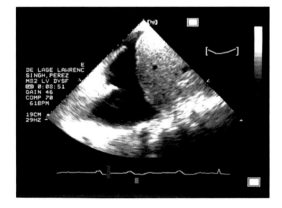

23. What view was used to obtain the image below?
    a. apical long axis
    b. apical four chamber
    c. subcostal
    d. apical two chamber

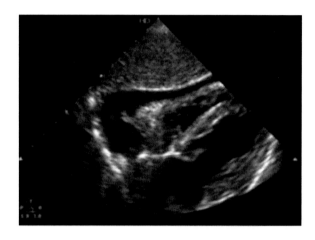

24. The following MV Doppler best describes:
    a. small pericardial effusion
    b. pericardial fat pad
    c. cardiac tamponade
    d. loculated pericardial effusion

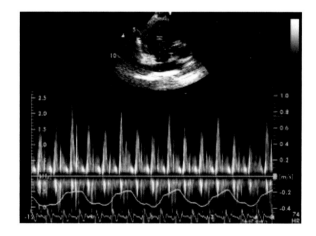

25. Diagnose the following M-mode in a patient with a large pericardial effusion:
    a. True prolapse
    b. Mitral stenosis
    c. Pseudo prolapse
    d. Mitral regurgitation

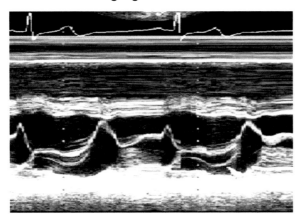

26. Diagnose the following 2D image:
    a. Small pericardial effusion
    b. Moderate pericardial effusion
    c. Pericardial fat pad
    d. Pleural effusion

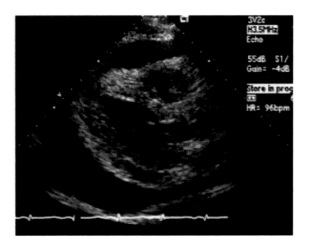

27. Clinical indications for cardiac tamponade that includes increased venous pressure, muffled heart sounds and hypotension best describes:
    a. Pulsus paradoxus
    b. Ewart's sign
    c. Beck's triad
    d. Paradoxic effusion

28. Diagnose the following image:
    a. Small pericardial effusion
    b. Fibrinous strands in the PE
    c. Mitral valve prolapse
    d. Pericardial cyst

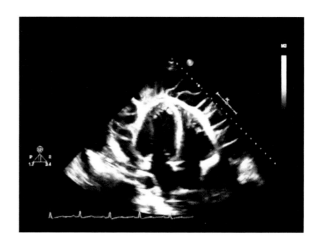

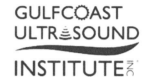

Section 5:

Systemic and Pulmonary Hypertensive Disease

Section 5: SYSTEMIC AND PULMONARY HYPERTENSIVE DISEASE

Objectives

Upon completion of this module you should be able to:

- State the difference between systemic and pulmonary hypertensive heart disease

- Outline echocardiographic imaging, M-mode and Doppler procedures used to evaluate systemic and pulmonary hypertensive heart disease

- Explain the etiologies for systemic and pulmonary hypertensive heart disease

- Apply quantitative methods for the determination of systemic and pulmonary hypertensive heart disease

- Identify the common echocardiographic findings associated with systemic and pulmonary hypertensive heart disease

SYSTEMIC and PULMONARY HYPERTENSIVE HEART DISEASE

SYSTEMIC HYPERTENSION

Hypertension occurs when the blood pressure rises higher than normal. There are no fixed rules regarding what is considered a normal blood pressure. According to the American Heart Association guidelines, a blood pressure reading that has been taken several times and on various occasions greater than 140/90 is considered abnormal while 120 – 139 systolic and 80 – 89 diastolic is considered "pre-hypertensive".

There are multiple conditions that may cause hypertension, but the primary factor is idiopathic increased peripheral resistance that results from vasoconstriction or narrowing of the peripheral vessels. Less common causes may be coarctation of the aorta, renal artery disease, and pheochromocytoma.

The most common response of the heart to chronic hypertension is concentric left ventricular hypertrophy. Left ventricular systolic function tends to be hyperdynamic, possibly causing a dynamic left ventricular outflow tract obstruction. Other cardiac findings associated with hypertensive heart disease include aortic valve sclerosis, dilatation of the aortic root, mitral annular calcification, left atrial enlargement, and atrial fibrillation.

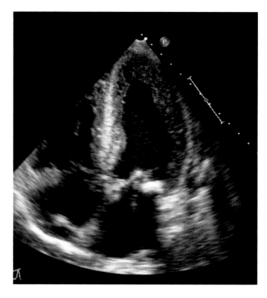

Apical Four Chamber LVH

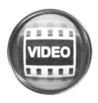

Play Video 5A:
Apical 4 chamber LVH

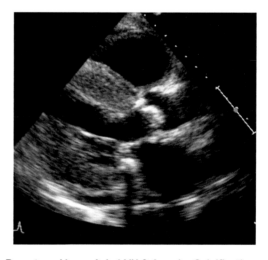

Parasternal Long Axis LVH & Annular Calcification

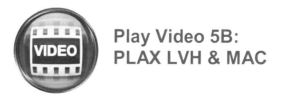

Play Video 5B:
PLAX LVH & MAC

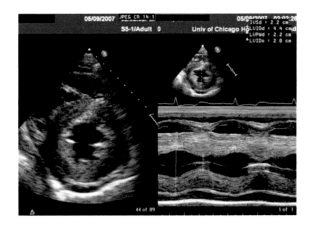

M-mode Left Ventricular Hypertrophy

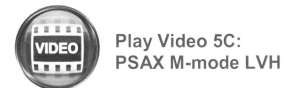

Play Video 5C:
PSAX M-mode LVH

Left ventricular diastolic function may also be compromised in patients with chronic hypertension due to abnormal relaxation of the cardiac muscle. Doppler indications of left ventricular diastolic dysfunction include reversal of the left ventricle E to A inflow velocity, prolonged left ventricle isovolumetric relaxation time, and prolonged mitral inflow deceleration time. In the event that congestive heart failure develops, or a hypertensive crisis occurs, the diastolic filling pattern may become pseudonormalized or restrictive.

When hypertrophy is present in a patient due to physical conditioning, abnormal E to A velocities are not usually seen.
The following parameters should be used for the echocardiographic assessment of systemic hypertension.

Assessment of Systemic Hypertension

- Left ventricular mass index
- Left ventricle cavity dimensions
- Left ventricle wall dimensions
- Left ventricle systolic function
- Left ventricle diastolic function
- Evaluation of LVOT to rule out obstruction
- Evaluation of the aorta for dissection, aneurysm and/or coarctation.

The methods commonly used to determine left ventricular systolic and diastolic function are discussed in chapter seven.

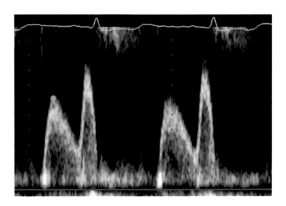

Reversal of E to A Inflow Velocity

156

PULMONARY HYPERTENSION

Pulmonary hypertension is the elevation of pulmonary arterial pressures higher than normal. The average mean pulmonary arterial pressure in a normal, supine, resting man at sea level, is approximately 9 - 18 mmHg.

Factors Causing Elevated Pulmonary Artery Pressures

- Elevation of the pulmonary capillary pressures.
- Elevation of the left atrial pressures.
- A decreased cross- sectional area of the total pulmonary vascular bed.
- A large increase in the blood flow from the pulmonary arteries.

Less important factors relating to pulmonary artery pressures are: pulmonary blood volume, viscosity of blood, bronchopulmonary arterial anastomosis, intrapulmonary pressure, and intrathoracic pressure.

Causes of elevated pulmonary capillary pressures and/ or left atrial pressures usually result from obstruction to the pulmonary venous blood flow. The obstruction can be as far distal as the left ventricle, or as proximal as the pulmonary veins. Increased left end diastolic pressures may result from left ventricular failure and, or hypertension. Mitral valve disease may cause increased left atrial pressure that can be transmitted to the pulmonary capillary bed since there are no valves between the left atrium and pulmonary veins. Other obstructions proximal to the mitral valve that may also cause pulmonary hypertension are: left atrial myxomas, cor triatriaum, congenital stenosis of the pulmonary veins, mediastinitis, and total anomalous pulmonary venous connections.

A decrease in the total cross-sectional area of the vascular bed causes an increase in resistance to pulmonary vascular flow. The pulmonary vascular bed needs to be reduced greater than 50% before a serious increase in pulmonary arterial pressure results. Increased resistance to pulmonary vascular flow may be caused by compression of pulmonary vessels by sarcoidosis, collagen vascular disease, COPD, and others.

Reduction within the vessels may occur due to miliary emboli, thrombosis of small pulmonary arteries, and from severe pulmonary hypertension.

Increased pulmonary blood flow is a rare cause of increased pulmonary artery pressures. The pulmonary bed has a large capacity for blood, so the amount of extra blood has to be great. Usually two conditions exist in order to create this problem. One is an overall reduction in cross-sectional area of the vascular bed, the second is an intracardiac septal defect with a large left to right shunt. Multiple septal defects are possible.

2-D and M-Mode Indications of Pulmonary Hypertension

- Decreased or flat/absent A wave of the pulmonic M-mode.
- A mid systolic notch, or "Flying W" on M-mode of pulmonic valve.
- Increased right ventricular systolic time interval.
- Increased right ventricle pre-ejection period to ejection time ratio.
- Enlarged right ventricle.
- Enlarged right atrium.
- Paradoxical septal motion.
- Right ventricular hypertrophy.
- Septal hypertrophy.
- Enlarged pulmonary artery
- Small to normal left ventricle
- Septal flattening causing a D-shaped left ventricle that persists during systole best seen in the PSAX view of the LV.

157

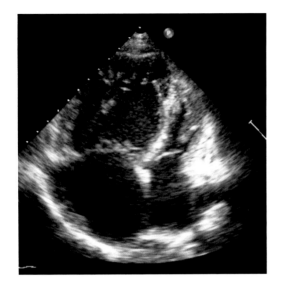

Apical Four Chamber of Enlarged RA/RV

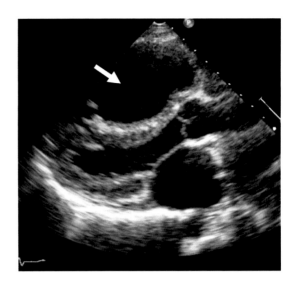

Parasternal Long Axis of RV volume overload

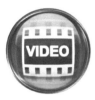

**Play Video 5D:
Apical 4 Chamber
enlarged RA/RV**

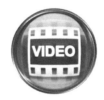

**Play Video 5F:
PLAX RV Volume
Overload PHTN**

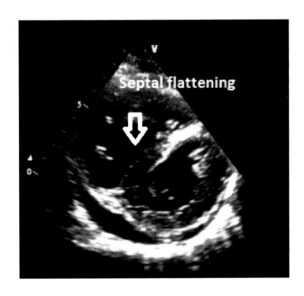

**Short Axis of Enlarged Right Ventricle with flattening of
IVS (arrow)**

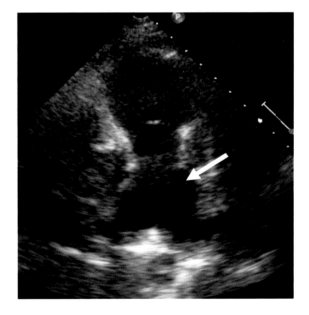

Enlarged pulmonary artery

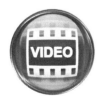

**Play Video 5E:
PSAX enlarged RV
with flattened IVS**

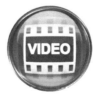

**Play Video 5G:
Enlarged pulmonary
artery PHTN**

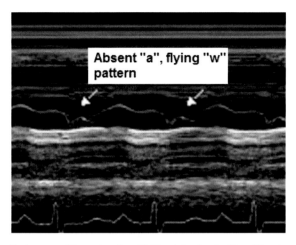

Pulmonary Hypertension RV Ventricular Outflow Tract

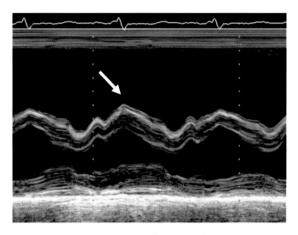

Paradoxical Septal Motion

Mid-systolic notching of the right ventricular outflow tract velocity

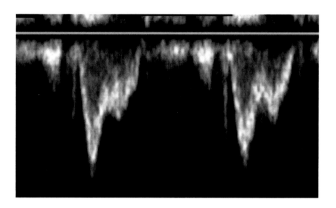

Absent A Flying "W" Pulmonic Valve M-mode

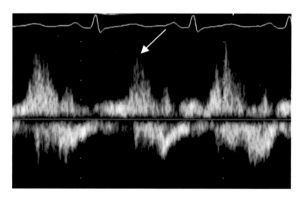

Hepatic Vein with Prominent Atrial Flow Reversal

Doppler Indications of Pulmonary Hypertension

- Pulmonic regurgitation
- Increased right ventricular systolic pressure of 30 mmHg or greater
- Acceleration time obtained from right ventricular outflow tract flow <120ms.
- Possible increased right ventricular isovolumetric relaxation time.
- Pulmonary acceleration time to ejection time ratio < 0.45 (abnormal)
- Prominent atrial flow reversal in the hepatic vein.

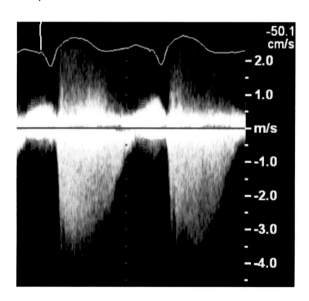

Increased Right Ventricular Systolic Pressure

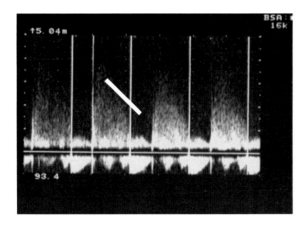

Flattened Pulmonic Valve Regurgitation, No Dip in CW Signa

Pulmonary artery pressure or right ventricular systolic pressure (**RVSP**) can be calculated by obtaining the peak velocity of the tricuspid regurgitation jet. The assumption is that PAP = RVSP in the absence of any significant pulmonary insufficiency or stenosis. Since the driving force of the tricuspid regurgitant jet is the RV systolic pressure it can be calculated using the Bernoulli equation in the following manner

PAP=4v^2(V=TR x PSV) + estimated RAP

However, since the regurgitant jet is not going into a vacuum but instead into the right atrium, the RA pressure needs to be estimated. Most labs typically add 5mmHg if it is assumed that the RA pressure is normal. The RA pressure is estimated by obtaining a view of the IVC and determining its size and collapsibility with respiration. In addition, a higher right atrial pressure can be assumed when the right atrium bulges towards the left atrium and the IVC and hepatic veins are dilated. This technique visualizes the IVC from the subcostal view at rest and during inspiration.

The American Society of Echocardiography (ASE) recommends that the overall size of the IVC is noted at the point where it passes through the diaphragm and enters the right atrium and collapsibility with

respiration is noted. This area is noted as just proximal to the junction of the hepatic veins. If the IVC is dilated and does not collapse >50% with changes in respiration, a higher right atrial pressure is suspected. The ASE caval diameter index is lower than some authors but also provides a more consistent location in which to measure the IVC diameter.

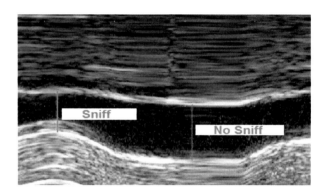

IVC Response indicating RA pressure is normal

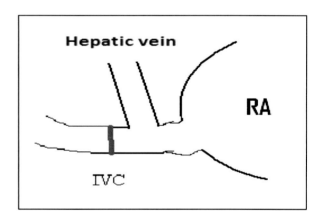

American Society of Echocardiography recommends the following caval index:

	IVC size	Collapse	Est. RAP
Normal	<2.1cm	>50%	0-5mmHg
Intermediate	<2.1cm >2.1cm	<50% >50%	5-10mmHg
High	>2.1cm	<50%	15mmHg

Source: The Echocardiographer's Pocket Reference (Reynolds)

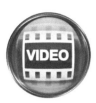

Play Video 5H: Severe Pulmonary Hypertension with dilated IVC and Hepatic Veins

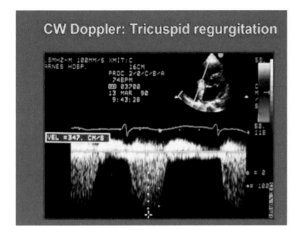

SPAP/PHTN Severity Scale	Values
Normal	18 – 25 mmHg
Mild	30 – 40 mmHg
Moderate	40 – 70 mmHg
Severe	>70 mmHg
Eisenmenger's	> 120 mmHg

Source: The Echocardiographer's Pocket Reference (Reynolds)

Pulmonary Embolus Echo findings:

- RV dilation
- Increase in pulmonary pressure
- Decrease in RV function
- Paradoxical septal motion
- Dilated pulmonary artery

The following example of how to calculate the **SPAP or RVSP** pressure is based on the information provided in the previous image.

1. The tricuspid regurgitant jet peak velocity is approximately 3.5 m/s.
2. The IVC was enlarged and did not collapse with respiration, therefore the RA pressure would be estimated at 15 mmHg.

Based on these findings, the **PAP** would be calculated as follows:

PAP/RVSP = $4V^2$ + 15 mmHg or
$4(3.5 \text{ m/s})^2$ + 15 mmHg
4(12.25) + 15
49 + 15
PAP = 64 mmHg

This method provides a reasonable non-invasive means of establishing PAP that correlates well with that obtained by catheterization. The one caveat to this method is to obtain a complete tricuspid regurgitant waveform and to carefully search for the highest velocity to avoid underestimation of the PAP. (*Otto, **The Practice of Clinical Echocardiography,** Saunders 2009*)

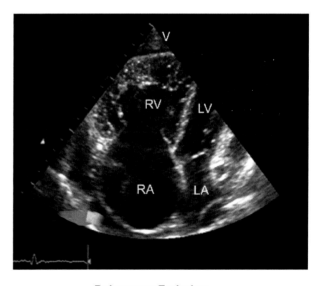

Pulmonary Embolus

SYSTEMIC AND PHTN HEART DISEASE QUIZ

1. The primary factor causing systemic hypertension is:
   a. aortic stenosis
   b. mitral stenosis
   c. increased peripheral resistance
   d. decreased peripheral resistance

2. Which of the following is NOT a common finding in chronic hypertension?
   a. concentric left ventricular hypertrophy
   b. aortic valve sclerosis
   c. aortic root enlargement
   d. decreased left ventricular systolic function

3. In patients with chronic SHTN the ascending aorta should be evaluated for which of the following?
   a. dilation or aneurysm
   b. dissection
   c. coarctation
   d. all of the above

4. Pulmonary artery pressure is considered elevated when it reaches which minimal level?
   a. > 12 mmHg
   b. > 20 mmHg
   c. > 30 mmHg
   d. > 50 mmHg

5. Which two conditions usually need to exist in order for the pulmonary bed to have an overload of blood flow?
   a. increase in the cross-sectional area of the vascular bed
   b. decrease in the cross-sectional area of the vascular bed
   c. septal defect with a large right to left shunt
   d. septal defect with a large left to right shunt
   e. a and c
   f. b and d

6. Assessment of patients with chronic hypertension should include which of the following?
   a. LV size for dilation
   b. LV Mass index
   c. LV systolic function
   d. LV diastolic function
   e. All of the above

7. Which one of the following is of less importance as a cause of elevated pulmonary artery pressure?
   a. viscosity of blood
   b. elevated pulmonary capillary pressure
   c. decreased cross-section area of the total pulmonary vascular bed
   d. a large increase in blood flow from the pulmonary arteries

8. The reduction in the pulmonary vascular bed needs to be greater than _____ before serious increases in pulmonary artery pressures are created.
   a. 20%
   b. 30%
   c. 50%
   d. 75%

9. Elevation of right heart pressures is indicated by all of the following 2D/M-mode findings EXCEPT:
   a. p aradoxical septal motion
   b. f lattened D shaped ventricular septum during systole
   c. absent "a" wave of the pulmonic M-mode
   d. D ecreased RV systolic time interval

10. Two-dimensional findings of pulmonary hypertension may be all of the following except:
    a. enlarged pulmonary artery
    b. enlarged right ventricle
    c. enlarged left ventricle
    d. paradoxical septal motion
    e. enlarged right atrium

11. Diagnose the following M-mode:
    a. Mitral valve prolapse
    b. Systolic anterior motion of the MV
    c. Pericardial effusion
    d. Left ventricular hypertrophy

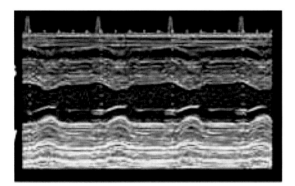

12. Diagnose the following Doppler image of the RVOT:
    a. Flying "W" of the Pulmonic valve
    b. Systolic anterior motion
    c. Mid-systolic notching of the RVOT
    d. Dilated pulmonary artery

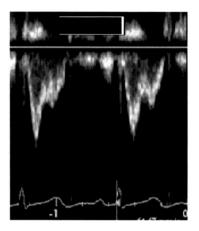

13. Diagnose the following 2D image:
    a. Mitral valve prolapse
    b. Increased right heart pressures
    c. Aortic valve stenosis
    d. Left ventricular dilatation

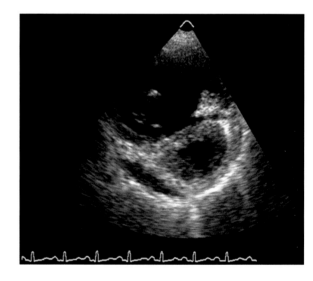

14. Patients in pulmonary hypertension may display this on the M-mode of the pulmonic valve?
    a. Absent "a" wave
    b. Increased "a" wave
    c. Flying "W" pattern
    d. Both a and c

15. Diagnose the following 2D image:
    a. Dilated RV
    b. Dilated LV
    c. Left ventricular hypertrophy
    d. Right ventricular hypertrophy

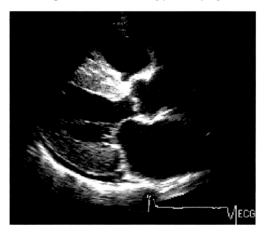

16. A pulmonary artery pressure of 50 mmHg indicates what degree of pulmonary hypertension:
    a. normal
    b. mild
    c. moderate
    d. severe

17. Diagnose the following Doppler image:
    a. decreased ventricular compliance
    b. mitral stenosis
    c. pseudonormalization
    d. systolic notching

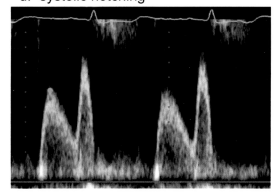

18. Determine the RVSP with the given information:

    TR velocity 2.8 m/sec

    a. 15 mmHg
    b. 36 mmHg
    c. 41 mmHg
    d. 56 mmHg

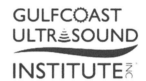

Section 6:

Cardiomyopathies

Section 6: CARDIOMYOPATHIES

Objectives

Upon completion of this module you should be able to:

- Identify the various types of cardiomyopathies
- State the etiologies of the various cardiomyopathies
- Differentiate on the echocardiogram the various types of cardiomyopathies from other diseases
- Apply quantitative measurements for the assessment of the hemodynamic effects caused by cardiomyopathies
- Implement echocardiographic methods used to identify and evaluate the various types of cardiomyopathies

Cardiomyopathies

Cardiomyopathies are diseases of the myocardium that are associated with cardiac dysfunction. In 1995 the World Health Organization/International Society and Federation of Cardiology Task Force suggested that the dominant physiologic cause or factor should dictate the classifications of cardiomyopathies.

CLASSIFICATION OF CARDIOMYOPATHIES

- Dilated cardiomyopathy
- Hypertrophic cardiomyopathy
- Restrictive cardiomyopathy
- Arrhythmogenic right ventricular cardiomyopathy

Hypertrophic

The hypertrophic cardiomyopathy is characterized by ventricular hypertrophy, especially affecting the interventricular septum. Typically, the left ventricle is involved, but one or both ventricles can be affected. Hypertrophic cardiomyopathy is usually an autosomal dominant inherited disease, but may be acquired in elderly, hypertensive patients. Symptoms with the inherited form commonly do not start until age thirty or older. The three major anatomic findings of a hypertrophic cardiomyopathy are: asymmetrical septal hypertrophy of the left ventricle, impaired diastolic left ventricular function, and preserved or hyperdynamic ventricular systolic function. Depending on the location of the septal hypertrophy, sub-aortic stenosis may be present.

Symptoms are variable depending on the severity or stage of the disease. Chest pain, syncope, fatigue, dyspnea, possible arrhythmia's, and a systolic ejection murmur may be heard with auscultation. Symptoms may occur only upon exertion, including sudden death.

The classic hypertrophic cardiomyopathy typically presents with asymmetrical septal hypertrophy, usually with some degree of myocardial thickening. Hypertrophic cardiomyopathies are categorized by patterns depending on the location of septal thickening.

PATTERNS OF HYPERTROPHIC CARDIOMYOPATHIES

- The hypertrophy is only in the **anterior interventricular septum (anteroseptal wall)** (90%).
- Hypertrophy involves the **basal septum** (15%)
- **Concentric hypertrophic** variant (1%)
- Hypertrophy involves the a**pical** region (1 – 3 %)

All of these patterns of hypertrophic cardiomyopathies have one feature in common, the thickness of the basal posterior wall is normal, or spared. Regardless of the location of the hypertrophy, the thickened area is at least 1.3 times greater than the basal posterior wall. The basal posterior wall region is located between the mitral valve and the papillary muscle. The apical region cardiomyopathy may be difficult to detect on the echocardiogram, but a contrast injection or inverted precordial T waves on EKG are clinical indications of its presence.

Left ventricular outflow tract obstruction, or subaortic stenosis, is the result of massive abnormal septal hypertrophy and, or abnormal placement of the mitral valve anteriorly and close to the interventricular septum. The abnormal mitral valve placement is caused by malpositioned papillary muscles that results in the tethering of the mitral valve. The left ventricular outflow tract obstruction is caused by the abnormal forward motion of the mitral valve and apposition of the anterior mitral leaflet with the thick interventricular septum causing a Venturi effect. The obstruction usually occurs in mid to late systole and the severity can change based on the loading conditions.

2-D FINDINGS WITH A HYPERTROPHIC CARDIOMYOPATHY

- Asymmetrical septal hypertrophy "ASH" in varying locations, but with sparing of the basal posterior wall.
- The thickened interventricular septum may be very echogenic or have a "ground glass" appearance or speckling.
- Systolic anterior motion "SAM "of the mitral valve. This is seen when there is an increased resting pressure gradient in the left ventricular outflow tract.
- Possible sclerosis of the aortic valve cusps.
- Possible contact lesion on the left ventricular side of the IVS.
- Possible mild calcification of the mitral valve annulus.

The "**ground glass**" appearance of the interventricular septum is caused by the abnormal cellular hypertrophy. The cells in the interventricular septum are shorter, wider, and arranged in a stellate configuration compared to the cells in a normal heart. This is referred to as "myocellular disarray".

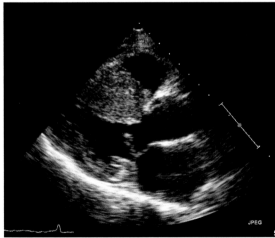

Long Axis Asymmetrical Septal Hypertrophy

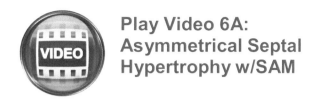

Play Video 6A: Asymmetrical Septal Hypertrophy w/SAM

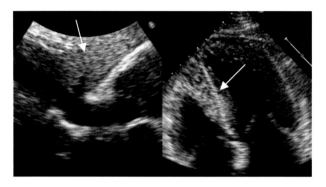

Thick IVS "Ground Glass" or Speckling (Liver-left, Septum-right)

If an outflow obstruction is present, it is considered a dynamic rather than a fixed obstruction since loading conditions affect its presence and severity.

Systolic anterior motion of the mitral valve can be caused by the abnormally positioned mitral valve, or in part to a vortices type effect created by the subaortic stenosis.

The M-mode patterns seen in the classic obstructive form of the hypertrophic cardiomyopathy can be helpful to document the various findings, but are not necessarily specific to that disease process alone.

M-mode Patterns with Hypertrophic Obstructive Cardiomyopathy

- Asymmetrical septal hypertrophy
- Increased echogenicity of the IVS

- Possible hypokinesis of the IVS (anteroseptal wall) with compensatory hyperkinetic posterior wall motion
- Possible LV cavity obliteration during systole.
- Systolic anterior motion of the mitral valve.
- Mid systolic notching or closure of the aortic valve.
- Possible left atrial enlargement.

When there is a left ventricular outflow tract obstruction, mid systolic notching of the aortic valve occurs due to the change in chamber pressure from the obstruction. Left atrial enlargement is typically mild to moderate and may be the result of the almost always present mitral regurgitation. Hypertrophic cardiomyopathies do not always create an outflow obstruction, this depends on the location of the hypertrophy and the volume status of the patient.

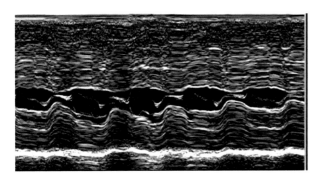

Asymmetrical Septal Hypertrophy

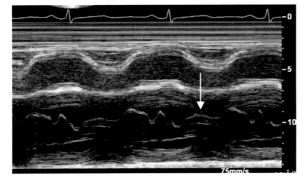

Systolic Anterior Motion

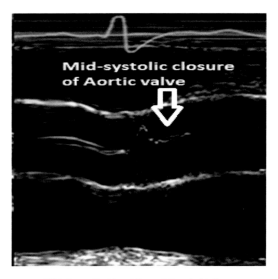

Mid-Systolic Notching of Aortic Valve

The Doppler exam is extremely helpful in locating the left ventricular outflow tract obstructive lesion. Color flow imaging may show an area of turbulence with high velocity flow. Parasternal views often help to demonstrate the obstructive lesion, but the apical views are best for Doppler interrogation.

Pulsed Doppler is helpful to locate the left ventricular outflow tract obstruction, but often continuous wave is needed to obtain the highest peak velocity. When the peak velocity of the outflow tract obstruction is obtained, a peak pressure gradient can be obtained by using the modified Bernoulli equation of $4V^2$. The left ventricular outflow tract waveform has a very distinct curve that relates to the left ventricular and aortic valve pressure gradients. The waveform is typically a late-peaking, high velocity, monophasic signal and is sometimes referred to as "dagger-shaped" in appearance. Gradients greater than 30 mmHg are considered to be significant.

Patients with systolic anterior motion usually have mild to moderate mitral regurgitation. Many times the spectral tracing from the mitral regurgitation is confused with the left ventricular outflow tract obstruction. Careful mapping and observation of the spectral tracing should help to alleviate this problem. The mitral regurgitation jet velocity can be used to help determine the severity of the

173

outflow obstruction by determining the LV to LA gradient and subtracting the systolic blood pressure

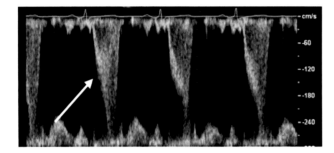

"Dagger-shaped" Doppler Signal LVOT

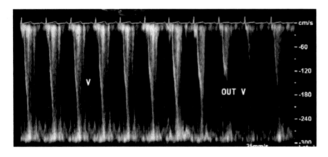

Valsalva provocation

LVOT gradient = LV pressure – systolic blood pressure.

Example...

Mitral regurgitant jet velocity = 6 m/s

LV-LA gradient = 4×6^2 = 144 mmHg.

LV pressure = 144 + 20 (LA pressure) =164 mmHg.

If the patient's blood pressure is 120/70
then
LVOT gradient = 164 – 120 = 44mmHg.

A small amount of aortic regurgitation may be seen in these patients. Right ventricular outflow tract obstruction may also occur, but is much less common.

One of the conditions associated with a hypertrophic cardiomyopathy is significantly impaired myocardial relaxation. The Doppler inflow velocity curve may show an abnormal E to A velocity with a reduced E velocity and an increased A velocity. The isovolumetric relaxation time and the deceleration time are prolonged. The inflow tracing should be obtained at the level of the mitral leaflet tips in the apical window

IVRT: 140msec
DT: 380msec
E/A Ratio: .69
E velocity: 77 CM/S
A velocity: 112 CM/S

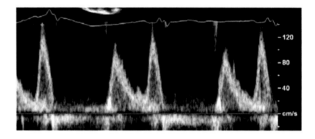

Abnormal Myocardial Relaxation

When a left ventricular outflow tract obstruction is only mildly evident, or not present during rest, provocative maneuvers should be performed to instigate or accentuate the obstruction. The Valsalva maneuver is performed by having the patient exhale and bear down. The straining phase of this maneuver decreases the pre-load which decreases left ventricle size and enhances the obstruction. This may be technically difficult to perform while trying to obtain accurate Doppler information.

Another method used to provoke or enhance an outflow tract obstruction is the use of amyl nitrate. The patient is instructed to inhale while the scan is performed. This should be done under the supervision of a physician. When amyl nitrate is inhaled it causes a short decrease in the pre-load and the afterload, resulting in an increase in the obstruction and a possible brief episode of tachycardia. During the period of obstruction, the highest velocities are

174

recorded. The patient should be monitored until the effects of the medication wear off.

Hypertrophic obstructive cardiomyopathy and concentric hypertrophic heart disease due to other abnormalities such as hypertension need to be carefully differentiated. Remember, patients with hypertrophic cardiomyopathy should have sparing of the posterior basal wall and left ventricular outflow obstructive patterns that demonstrate a late-peaking systolic signal.

Patients with left ventricular hypertrophy may have a similar appearance of a small left ventricle with some cavity obliteration, a hyperdynamic left ventricle, and possibly an intracavitary gradient with late peaking velocities, but the location and timing of the obstructions are different and the basal posterior wall will not be spared.

Occasionally, patients have both hypertrophic obstructive cardiomyopathy and aortic stenosis. High pulse repetition frequency Doppler may help to locate and differentiate each high velocity jet and give some indication as to the severity of both.

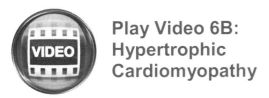

Play Video 6B: Hypertrophic Cardiomyopathy

DILATED CARDIOMYOPATHY

The characteristic findings of the dilated or congestive cardiomyopathy are dilatation of the left ventricle with moderate to marked enlargement of the end-systolic and end-diastolic dimensions, and decreased global systolic function. All of the cardiac chambers may become involved. Causes are variable for this disease and may be idiopathic.

Possible Etiologies for Dilated Cardiomyopathy

- Idiopathic
- Ischemic
- AIDS
- Chemotherapeutic agents
- Toxic
- Alcohol (most common secondary cause)
- Medications
- Radiation
- Pre and post-partum
- Infections
- Viral
- Chagas' disease
- Systemic hypertension
- Inherited diseases/congenital
- Sickle cell anemia
- Duchenne's muscular dystrophy
- Non-compaction

The etiology of a dilated cardiomyopathy is typically difficult to determine with echocardiography, except in the case of Chagas' heart disease. Chagas' disease is rare in North America, but endemic in South and Central America. Patients' with a dilated cardiomyopathy related to Chagas' disease have a left ventricular aneurysm that may minimally involve the interventricular septum. If endomyocardial fibrosis due to Chagas' disease occurs, there may be obliteration of the ventricle which is small, and atrial enlargement with regurgitation.

Ischemia is also a cause of a dilated cardiomyopathy. This occurs due to severe cardiac insufficiency that results in pump failure. Progressive heart failure results rather than angina and infarction. Coronary artery spasm and coronary embolism may also cause an ischemic type dilated cardiomyopathy.

At autopsy, a heart with a dilated cardiomyopathy is typically enlarged and heavier than the normal heart even though the walls usually appear normal or thin. The ventricular contractility is impaired resulting in a reduced cardiac output and elevated end-diastolic pressures due to the left ventricular volume overload.

Since the left ventricle is enlarged, the mitral valve annulus is dilated and mild to moderate mitral regurgitation is often present. When there is chronic mitral regurgitation, typically mild to moderate left atrial enlargement occurs. Left atrial pressures are often increased leading to pulmonary hypertension. Left ventricle diastolic dysfunction may occur and may be an important prognostic indicator. Clinically, patients present with symptoms of heart failure. Dyspnea, chest pain, peripheral edema, and arrhythmias are common.

The 2-D exam shows marked chamber enlargement usually evident in the left ventricle, however there is commonly some degree of enlargement in all chambers. There is a marked increased distance between the anterior mitral leaflet tip in diastole and the interventricular septum, or increased e-point to septal separation (EPSS). The walls of the heart may be mildly hypertrophied, but usually are normal or thin. There is an obvious decrease in overall cardiac wall motion. The walls of the left ventricle are globally hypokinetic with possible areas of akinesis or dyskinesis. An absence of systolic thickening will be noted if a wall motion abnormality is present. If a wall motion abnormality is present, conditions are right for mural thrombus to occur. Careful scanning of these areas is necessary since thrombus can often be similar in echo texture as the heart walls. An ejection fraction that is 35% or less is considered a good condition for clot formation. Left ventricular function should be evaluated. Measurements include the ejection fraction, fractional shortening, cardiac output, and stroke volume. Ventricular function is an important factor in the prediction of the outcome for the patient and may help with medical treatment, as well as for consideration for heart transplant.

Dilated cardiomyopathy is the primary reason for heart transplant.

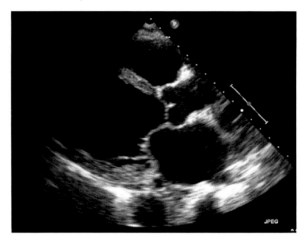

Parasternal Long Axis of dilated left heart

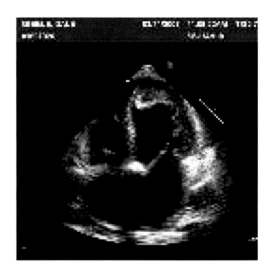

Apical 4C of mural thrombus

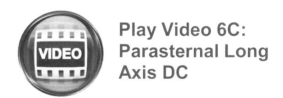

Play Video 6C: Parasternal Long Axis DC

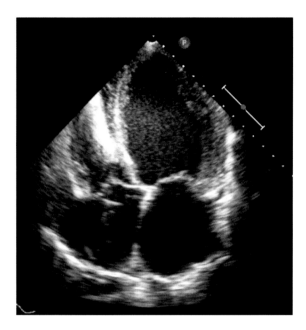

Dilated Cardiomyopathy Apical Four Chamber

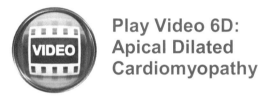

Play Video 6D: Apical Dilated Cardiomyopathy

M-mode findings are easily identified in patients with a dilated cardiomyopathy. Chamber sizes will be increased, especially the left ventricle. M-mode parameters of left ventricular function will be reduced including: ejection fraction, shortening fraction, and cardiac output. There will be at least mild to moderate enlargement of the right ventricle, right atrium, and left atrium. Wall motion will be abnormal and variable.

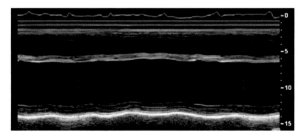

M-mode Dilated Cardiomyopathy

The M-mode tracing of the mitral valve may demonstrate several features. The EPSS or E point to septal separation will be markedly increased, an indication of poor left ventricle

function and dilatation. There will be a "double-diamond" appearance of the mitral valve due to the left ventricular enlargement that results in an increased distance between the valve and heart wall. The P-R A-C interval on the mitral valve may be abnormal. There may be a "B" bump or notch on the mitral valve tracing indicating elevated left ventricular end diastolic pressure.

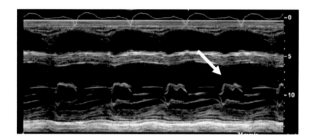

Mitral Valve M-mode "Double Diamond" and Increased EPSS

The aortic root appears immobile or decreased in mobility. This is due to the reduced left atrial filling and emptying that results from the low cardiac output. The aortic cusps may appear sloped in systole, also due to the low output state.

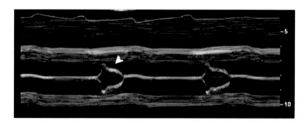

Gradual/Early closure of the Aortic Valve in low output

The Doppler exam may demonstrate multiple hemodynamic events. There is almost always some degree of valvular regurgitation, especially involving the mitral and tricuspid valves. If present, the severity can be evaluated with pulsed or continuous wave Doppler and/or Color flow imaging. If tricuspid regurgitation is present, the pulmonary artery pressure should be evaluated by obtaining the tricuspid regurgitation jet peak velocity and applying it to the equation $RVSP = 4V^2 + RAP$.

The pulmonary artery pressure may be an important factor in the prognosis of the patient. Tricuspid regurgitation velocities that are greater than 3 m/s are associated with a higher mortality rate, more frequent hospitalization, and higher occurrences of heart failure.

It is common for high tricuspid velocities to coincide with restrictive diastolic filling patterns and both together help to indicate the patients' that are at a higher risk for heart failure and death. Mild aortic regurgitation may be present, as well as mild to moderate pulmonic regurgitation.

Mitral inflow patterns can help to determine left ventricular filling pressures and diastolic function. The mitral inflow tracing should be obtained at, or slightly past the leaflet tips. An impaired relaxation pattern may be seen in patients having close to normal cardiac output and stroke volume, while those who have more advanced disease with a decreased stroke volume, typically have a restrictive diastolic filling pattern. The restrictive filling pattern results from an increase in left ventricular filling pressures and decreased compliance.

The deceleration time can be a valuable indicator in the prognosis of patients with a dilated cardiomyopathy. A shortened deceleration time suggests a poor prognosis. If a patient responds positively to treatment for heart failure, diastolic filling may become less restrictive and the deceleration time increases. The reversal of this pattern is a good indicator of survival and improvement. When the restrictive pattern does not change after therapy, the prognosis is poor. The timing of the diastolic filling should be coordinated properly with the PR interval.

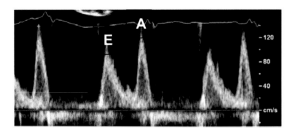

Impaired Relaxation Pattern

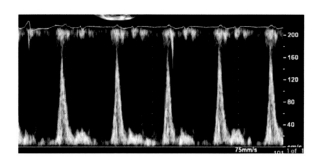

Restrictive Diastolic Filling Pattern

The mitral regurgitation jet may have a slow rise rate of velocity indicating a reduction in the rate of increase in the left ventricle pressure in early systole. This is the dP/dt. The dP/dt is a reflection of the rate of pressure decline from the maximum point to the opening of the mitral valve.

RESTRICTIVE CARDIOMYOPATHY

Restrictive cardiomyopathy occurs when stiffening of the myocardium results in restricted filling of the ventricles.

Etiologies of restrictive cardiomyopathy
- Amyloidosis (most common)
- Hemochromatosis
- Sarcoidosis
- Glycogen storage diseases
- Hypereosinophilic syndrome or Loeffler's endocarditis (rare).
- Hurler's syndrome (rare)
- Neuromuscular disease (rare)
- Metastatic tumor involvement (rare)
- Idiopathic
- Diabetic cardiomyopathy

Patients usually present with symptoms of heart failure that result from the increased left ventricular end diastolic pressure and the lack of ability to increase cardiac output due to the impaired diastolic filling. Diagnosis of a restrictive cardiomyopathy can be difficult and often other means such as endocardial biopsy may be necessary. The "square root" sign or configuration is a hemodynamic feature seen in the ventricular

178

diastolic pressure tracing. The 2-D exam may show increased echogenicity or speckling of the myocardium which may indicate the degree of involvement. The left ventricular chamber size is normal with normal to thickened walls. Systolic function is preserved initially, but diastolic function is not. Often the right ventricular free wall is hypertrophied. Biatrial enlargement may be a striking finding due to the impaired ventricular filling. A small to moderate pericardial and/or pleural effusion may be present. The inferior vena cava and hepatic veins are often dilated and do not vary in size with respiration.

Play Video 6E: Restrictive Cardiomyopathy/ Amyloid

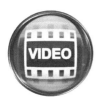

Play Video 6F: Dilated Inferior Vena Cava

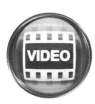

Play Video 6G: Enlarged RA, Dilated IVC

M-mode findings generally demonstrate normal to small left and right ventricles, dilated atria, and right ventricular hypertrophy.

Doppler findings in a restrictive cardiomyopathy often demonstrate mild to moderate mitral and tricuspid regurgitation. Pulmonary hypertension may be confirmed based on the findings of time to peak velocity of the pulmonary artery and the estimate of the right atrial pressure using the tricuspid regurgitation jet. The evaluation of left ventricular diastolic function may be difficult depending on the stage at which the cardiomyopathy is found. In the early phase of the disease, the left ventricle inflow pattern may show a reduced E to A velocity suggesting impaired diastolic relaxation of the left ventricle. Progression of the disease results in increased left atrial pressures and continued reduced left ventricular compliance. This results in a pseudonormalized E to A pattern. In the advanced stage of the restrictive cardio-myopathy, as the left ventricular compliance continues to decrease, the E velocity becomes much higher than the A. The E to A ratio is significantly increased.

Doppler Findings in Restrictive Cardiomyopathy

Increased mitral E velocity > 1m/s
Increased tricuspid E velocity >0.7 m/s
Decreased mitral A velocity <0.5 m/s
Decreased tricuspid A velocity <0.3 m/s
Increased E to A ratio ≥ 2.0
Decreased isovolumetric relaxation time <70msec
Decreased A duration

Source: The Echo Manual (Oh et al.)

The flow in the hepatic vein may show a prominent reversal with atrial contraction that may be followed by rapid filling in systole.

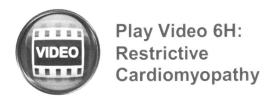

Play Video 6H: Restrictive Cardiomyopathy

ARRHYTHMOGENIC RIGHT VENTRICULARCARDIOMYOPATHY

This type of cardiomyopathy may also be referred to as RV dysplasia. The dysplasia is caused by replacement of the myocardium in the RV with fatty and fibrous tissue. Clinical indications are arrhythmia, heart murmur, congestive heart failure, and sudden death. The right ventricle is dilated and contracts poorly, RV systolic pressure may be low due to pump failure, and LV dilatation and dysfunction may be present.

TAKOTSUBO CARDIOMYOPATHY

Also known as broken heart syndrome, this type of cardiomyopathy presents as acute heart failure due to sudden, intense emotional or physical stress. Signs and symptoms for this cardiomyopathy may include: chest pain, ST segment elevation or T wave inversion, and elevated cardiac enzyme levels. Typically normal coronary anatomy will be demonstrated on coronary angiogram. Echocardiographic findings include: reduced EF%, apical wall motion abnormality (apical ballooning), and possible apical thrombus.

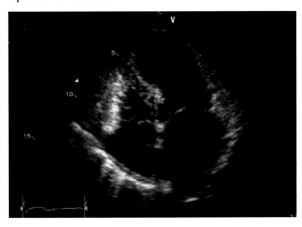

Apical ballooning in patient with Takotsubo Cardiomyopathy

SYSTEMIC DISEASES AFFECTING THE HEART

There are many heart conditions that can result from systemic diseases. The heart is often affected well after the disease has been diagnosed and progressed through the various other systems.

Marfan's syndrome is an inherited disorder of the connective tissue which is inherited as an autosomal dominant trait. This disease is characterized by a defective gene coding for fibrillin that partly makes up microfibrils which are important structures in elastic fibers. This results in possible abnormalities in the musculoskeletal, ocular and cardiovascular systems that can be of varying degrees. Marfan's patients tend to be taller than average for age and their arm span exceeds their height. Several other conditions may affect Marfan's patients such as: long, thin digits, pectus carinatum or outward displacement of the sternum, or pectus excavatum or inward displacement. Joints may be hyperextensible with backward curvature of the legs and knees, and flat feet, kyphosis, and hernias are common. Ocular problems such as: dislocation of the lens, high grade myopia, and retinal detachment may occur.

In relation to the cardiovascular system, Marfan's patients may have dilated arteries, aneurysms and or rupture of peripheral arteries. The anterior mitral leaflet may be redundant.

On the echocardiogram the characteristic findings of Marfan's syndrome are a dilated aortic root, annulus, and/or sinuses of Valsalva and possibly the ascending aorta. The sinotubular junction will be ill-defined. When the aortic annulus is dilated aortic regurgitation is probable. This in turn leads to a left ventricular volume overload. Aortic dissection is a frequent complication and may occur in patients with a mild to moderately dilated aorta. Aortic root diameters of greater than 55mm are considered high risk for spontaneous rupture and prophylactic aortic root replacement may be performed

Lupus erythematosus is one of the most common collagen diseases. It can affect the endocardium, myocardium, and pericardium, together or separately. One of the most well-known cardiac complications in systemic lupus is Libman-Sachs endocarditis. This occurs in approximately 50% of cases. Patients with Libman-Sachs endocarditis have verrucous lesions in the endocardium. These are wart-like and vary in size and number from a pinhead to 3-4mm.

The verrucae are made up of degenerating valve tissue and fibrosis. The lesions can form anywhere on the endocardial surface, but are most often found on the atrioventricular valve angles and on the underside of the mitral valve base. They usually do not get large enough to interfere with the valves.

The myocardium may be involved in patients with Lupus due to the deposits of fibrinoid material between the myocardial cells. These patients may have arteritis, periarteritis, and arrhythmia's. Cardiac enlargement often occurs most likely secondary to hypertension, renal disease, small vessel arteritis, and other factors. Pericarditis is a common cardiac lesion found with lupus. Large pericardial effusions either clear or bloody may be found and are most likely secondary to the acute inflammatory process of the disease.

Systemic sclerosis or scleroderma is another collagen disease that can affect the heart. It is a chronic disease of unknown origin that is characterized by diffuse fibrosis, vascular abnormalities of the skin, internal organs, and degenerative changes. This disease can vary in the degree of severity and the progression. If the heart is involved, the endocardium, myocardium, and pericardium may be affected. The myocardium is most often involved.

Patients with cardiac involvement of scleroderma have replacement of cardiac muscle with connective tissue. This may be marked or just patchy replacement.
Rheumatoid arthritis may result in cardiac complications. Subcutaneous nodules may form in the pericardium, myocardium, or epicardium. Rheumatoid nodules may involve valves, but do not usually affect the valve function.

Neuromuscular disorders such as muscular dystrophies can cause heart failure in two ways. The weakness of the muscles and the thoracic deformity. These may cause ventricular problems, typically right ventricular failure. Duchenne's muscular dystrophy has an onset at an early age and progresses rapidly. This is seen primarily in males. Heart failure is common with Duchenne's muscular dystrophy. Atrophy and fibrosis of the myocardium may occur resulting in cardiomyopathy.

Hematologic disorders can affect the heart. Chronic hemolytic anemias often cause severe cardiomegaly and heart failure due to the excessive deposits of iron in the myocardium.

Sickle cell anemia may cause a cardiomyopathy as a result of the physio chemical changes occurring with the blood cells. These patients may have a tendency toward thrombosis, pulmonary emboli, and other occlusive vascular lesions.

Thalassemia is another hemolytic anemia which may have cardiac involvement.

Endocrine and metabolic disorders may affect the heart. There are numerous types of these disorders that may affect the heart, but the more common ones will be discussed.

Abnormal amounts of thyroid hormones can affect the heart. **Thyrotoxicosis** or excessive thyroid hormone can have numerous cardiovascular implications. Several conditions produce excessive thyroid hormone including Grave's disease, Plummer's disease, toxic adenoma, some stages of Hashimoto's thyroiditis, and excessive exogenous thyroid administration. Clinically, patients have tachycardia, bounding pulses, irregular heartbeat, and heart failure. Arrhythmia's and congestive heart failure are the major clinical problems in thyrotoxicosis, but cardiac enlargement and hypertrophy may be long term effects. Patients often have the following: an increased heart rate, stroke volume, cardiac output, mean left ventricular systolic ejection rate, mean left ventricular circumferential shortening rate, coronary blood flow, and myocardial oxygen consumption.

Decreased thyroid hormone production, **hypothyroidism,** or **myxedema**, are conditions that result in decreased metabolic rates. These occur more often in older children and adults. Indications of cardiac involvement are a significantly reduced resting cardiac output. Clinically, these patients often have fatigue, dyspnea, orthopnea, and possible bradycardia. Cardiomegaly may result due to pericardial effusion. The effusion may have a "gold paint" appearance due to the high cholesterol content if pericardiocentesis is performed.

Acromegaly is caused by hypersecretion of growth hormones by a pituitary adenoma. This results in increased growth in the bones. Overgrowth of the jaw is also noted. The hands and feet are widened and the heart and kidneys may also be enlarged. Cardiomegaly often occurs past the fifth decade of life. Hypertension and atherosclerosis are common. Cushing's disease also results in pituitary hypersecretions.

CARDIOMYOPATHIES QUIZ

1. Which one of the following cardiomyopathies is often a result of an autosomal dominant inherited disease?
   a. dilated cardiomyopathy
   b. congestive cardiomyopathy
   c. hypertrophic cardiomyopathy
   d. restrictive cardiomyopathy

2. Symptoms associated with this cardiomyopathy may only be experienced during exercise?
   a. dilated
   b. infiltrative
   c. congestive
   d. hypertrophic

3. Which of the following is NOT a finding with a classic hypertrophic obstructive cardiomyopathy?
   a. asymmetrical septal hypertrophy
   b. systolic anterior motion
   c. sub-aortic stenosis
   d. left ventricular enlargement

4. The most common area affected in hypertrophic cardiomyopathy is:
   a. apical region
   b. anterior septal region
   c. concentric hypertrophy
   d. mid ventricular region

5. Which type of hypertrophic cardiomyopathy can cause LVOT obstruction?
   a. apical region
   b. anterior septal hypertrophy
   c. concentric hypertrophy
   d. mid ventricular region

6. The one finding that all types of hypertrophic cardiomyopathies have in common is:
   a. sub-aortic stenosis
   b. systolic anterior motion
   c. normal thickness of the basal posterior (inferolateral) left ventricle wall
   d. asymmetrical septal hypertrophy

7. The speckling or increased in echogenicity of the interventricular septum in the hypertrophic cardiomyopathy may also be referred to as the _____ appearance?
   a. "hockey stick"
   b. "crushed ice"
   c. "ground glass"
   d. "water balloon"

8. When should provocative maneuvers be performed on a patient with hypertrophic cardiomyopathy?
   a. when LVOT obstruction is severe
   b. when LVOT obstruction is moderate
   c. when LVOT obstruction is mildly evident at rest
   d. provocative maneuvers should never be performed

9. When hypertrophic obstructive cardiomyopathy is present, the outflow obstruction is considered to be:
   a. dynamic
   b. fixed
   c. alternating
   d. none of the above

10. Which one of the following is NOT a possible finding with a hypertrophic cardiomyopathy?
    a. aortic valve sclerosis
    b. mid systolic notching of the aortic valve
    c. a contact lesion on the left ventricular side of the interventricular septum
    d. a contact lesion on the right ventricular side of the interventricular septum

183

11. The M-mode tracing of the MV demonstrates:
    a. systolic anterior motion
    b. mid-systolic notching
    c. dilated left atrium
    d. "hockey stick" appearance

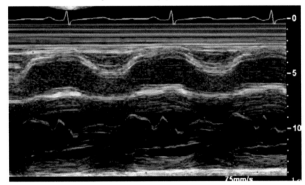

12. Asymmetrical septal hypertrophy is considered when the thickened area of the interventricular septum is _____ times thicker than the basal posterior wall.
    a. 5
    b. 3
    c. 2
    d. 1.3

13. When trying to obtain the peak gradient on a patient with a hypertrophic obstructive cardiomyopathy, the Doppler should be directed:
    a. distal to the aortic valve
    b. into the left ventricular outflow tract
    c. into the left ventricular inflow tract
    d. into the right ventricular outflow tract

14. Which of the following is NOT a typical finding in a hypertrophic cardiomyopathy?
    a. asymmetrical septal hypertrophy
    b. abnormal left ventricular systolic function
    c. normal left ventricular systolic function
    d. impaired left ventricular diastolic function

15. When diastolic dysfunction is present the Doppler inflow tracing will reveal:
    a. reduced E velocity
    b. Increased A velocity
    c. prolonged IVRT and deceleration time
    d. all of the above

16. The presence of outflow obstruction depends on:
    a. location of hypertrophy
    b. presence of MR
    c. volume status of patient
    d. presence of AS
    e. a & c
    f. a & b

17. The primary differentiating characteristic between hypertrophic cardiomyopathy and LV hypertrophy is:
    a. late peaking systolic velocity with HOCM only
    b. late peaking systolic velocity with LVH only
    c. sparing of the basal LVPW with HOCM only
    d. sparing of the basal LVPW with LVH only

18. Which of the following causes of a dilated or congestive cardiomyopathy can be detected on echocardiography?
    a. Chagas' disease
    b. alcoholic cardiomyopathy
    c. diabetic cardiomyopathy
    d. postpartum cardiomyopathy

19. What is the finding with Chagas' disease that helps to identify it as the cause of a dilated cardiomyopathy?
    a. dilated left ventricle
    b. mitral regurgitation
    c. left ventricle aneurysm
    d. dilated right ventricle

20. Which of the following is NOT a typical M-mode finding with a dilated cardiomyopathy?
    a. systolic anterior motion
    b. increased EPSS
    c. "double diamond" mitral valve
    d. immobile aortic root

21. Which of the following is NOT a finding with a dilated cardiomyopathy?
    a. increased cardiac output
    b. decreased cardiac output
    c. elevated end-diastolic pressure
    d. mitral regurgitation

22. An important factor to determine the prognosis of a patient with a dilated cardiomyopathy is:
    a. pulmonary artery pressure
    b. diastolic function
    c. LV filling patterns
    d. all of the above

23. Ejection fractions that are _____ or less are considered good conditions for clot formation?
    a. 40%
    b. 50%
    c. 60%
    d. 35%

24. Immobility of the aortic root is caused by:
    a. reduced left atrial emptying and filling
    b. increased left atrial emptying and filling
    c. reduced aortic valve filling
    d. mitral regurgitation

25. Sloping (gradual closure) of the aortic cusp is a finding commonly seen with:
    a. HOCM
    b. dilated cardiomyopathy
    c. restrictive cardiomyopathy
    d. lupus erythematosus

26. Which of the following is NOT a probable Doppler finding with a dilated cardiomyopathy?
    a. mitral regurgitation
    b. tricuspid regurgitation
    c. pulmonic stenosis
    d. pulmonic regurgitation

27. The most common cause of a restrictive cardiomyopathy is:
    a. hemochromatosis
    b. amyloidosis
    c. sarcoidosis
    d. Hurler's syndrome

28. In the advanced stage of a restrictive cardiomyopathy the E to A pattern will reveal:
    a. normal E to A velocity
    b. reduced E to A velocity
    c. Pseudonormal E to A pattern
    d. E to A significantly increased

29. Because of the infiltrative process of the restrictive cardiomyopathy the myocardium may appear:
    a. decreased in echogenicity
    b. increased in echogenicity
    c. no change in echogenicity
    d. thinned

30. Which of the following is NOT a probable finding with a restrictive cardiomyopathy?
    a. bilateral atrial enlargement
    b. small to moderate pericardial effusion
    c. normal diastolic function
    d. right ventricular hypertrophy

31. The following M-mode tracing indicates:
    a. a dilated left ventricle
    b. asymmetrical septal hypertrophy
    c. paradoxical septal motion
    d. right ventricular volume overload

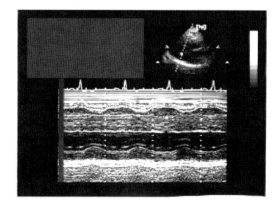

32. The Doppler tracing below is suggestive of:
    a. normal LV inflow
    b. restrictive diastolic filling
    c. impaired relaxation
    d. a hypertrophic cardiomyopathy

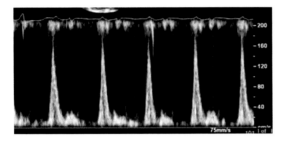

33. The Doppler tracing below is associated with which type of condition?
    a. diastolic filling
    b. Marfan's disease
    c. LVOT obstruction
    d. impaired relaxation

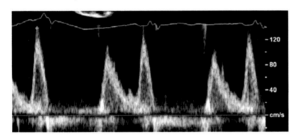

34. The best diagnosis for the following M-mode tracing is a (an):
    a. increased EPSS
    b. decreased E-F slope
    c. increased DE excursion
    d. decreased Isovolumetric relaxation time

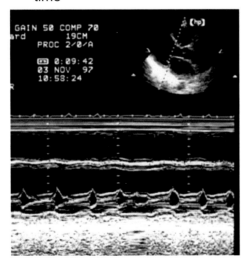

35. An aortic root diameter greater than _____ is considered high risk for spontaneous rupture:
    a. 45mm
    b. 40mm
    c. 37mm
    d. 55mm

36. One of the most well-known cardiac complications in patients with lupus erythematosus is:
    a. pleural effusion
    b. Libman-Sach's endocarditis
    c. Lambl's excrescences
    d. left ventricular thrombus

37. The part of the heart <u>most often</u> affected in patients with scleroderma is the:
    a. pericardium
    b. myocardium
    c. endocardium
    d. atrioventricular valves

38. Heart failure due to excessive deposits of iron in the myocardium is associated with:
    a. rheumatoid arthritis
    b. endocrine and metabolic disorder
    c. hematologic disorders
    d. neuromuscular disorders

39. The two ways in which muscular dystrophies cause heart failure are:
    a. muscle weakness
    b. mitral stenosis
    c. thoracic deformity
    d. left atrial enlargement
    e. a and c
    f. b and d
    g. a and d

40. Which of the following findings are not associated with lupus erythematosus.
    a. cardiac enlargement
    b. dilated aortic root
    c. pericarditis
    d. large pericardial effusion

41. The most common secondary cause of a dilated cardiomyopathy is:
    a. Alcohol
    b. Illicit drugs
    c. Environmental toxins
    d. Gluten

42. Diagnose the following 2D image:
    a. HOCM
    b. Mitral valve prolapse
    c. Amyloidosis
    d. Aortic stenosis

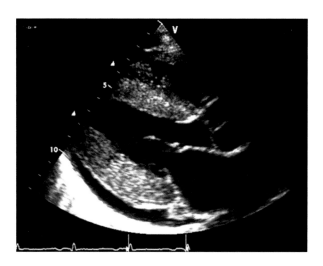

43. Diagnose the following image:
    a. HOCM
    b. Pericardial effusion
    c. Dilated CM
    d. Restrictive CM

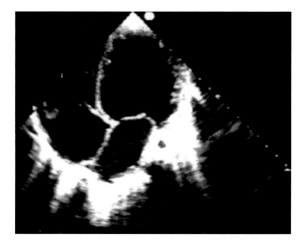

44. If "smoke" is seen in the LV apex, what should be the concern?
    a. Aortic stenosis
    b. Mitral valve prolapse
    c. Apical thrombus
    d. Vegetation on the MV

45. A LVOT gradient greater than _____ is considered to be significant.
    a. 15 mmHg
    b. 20 mmHg
    c. 25 mmHg
    d. 30 mmHg

46. A cardiomyopathy brought on by emotion or physical stress that causes apical ballooning of the LV best describes:
    a. Dilated CM
    b. HOCM
    c. Arrhythmogenic RV CM
    d. Takotsubo CM

Section 7:

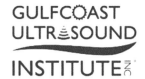

Ventricular Function

Section 7: VENTRICULAR FUNCTION

Objectives

Upon completion of this module you should be able to:

- Identify wall motion abnormalities on the echocardiogram

- Recognize the echocardiographic findings associated with coronary artery disease

- List the effects of coronary artery disease on diastolic function

- Apply quantitative methods for the evaluation of left ventricular function

- State the various complications associated with coronary artery disease

VENTRICULAR FUNCTION

WALL MOTION ABNORMALITIES

Ischemia is a local and temporary deficiency of blood supply due to obstruction of the circulation to a part of the body. When the heart muscle is involved, either temporary or permanent damage to the muscle may result. The amount of damage depends on the length of time the event lasts and the severity of the obstruction. A myocardial infarction most commonly results from the obstruction of the coronary artery by a thrombus, atherosclerosis, or vasospasm. When blood flow to the heart muscle is obstructed, tissue necrosis occurs resulting in death of that tissue. When intervention is quick and successful, tissue can be saved.

Obstruction of the artery greater than 70% in cross-sectional area is inadequate for myocardial demand during exercise, stress, or pharma- cological intervention. Motion abnormalities should be noted at this time, but at rest if no prior myocardial infarction has occurred, the wall motion appears normal. Sometimes patients with an acute myocardial infarction receiving thrombolytic therapy (or patients with prolonged ischemia) may have what is referred to as stunned tissues. Stunned tissue is a wall motion abnormality that lasts for 24-72 hours, but irreversible damage has not occurred. Cardiac tissue may appear abnormal, but may be hibernating during rest. Hibernating tissue begins to function with reperfusion through exercise or medication.

- **Hypokinesis** - reduced wall motion with reduced systolic thickening.

- **Akinesis** - absent inward wall motion and systolic thickening less than 10%.
- **Dyskinesis** - paradoxical motion of the ventricular segment during systole and no systolic thickening.
- **Aneurysmal-** thinned and scarred segment with diastolic deformation. At risk for rupture.

Anatomy of the coronary arteries may vary slightly among patients, but is typically similar. The right and left coronary arteries arise from their respective sinus of Valsalva. The left coronary artery divides into the left anterior descending artery and the circumflex artery. The right coronary artery gives rise to the posterior descending artery. Right dominant coronary artery circulation occurs in approximately 80% of patients.

Approximately 20% of patients have left dominant coronary artery circulation where the circumflex artery gives rise to the posterior descending artery. From these main arteries, smaller arteries arise and feed the various parts of the heart.

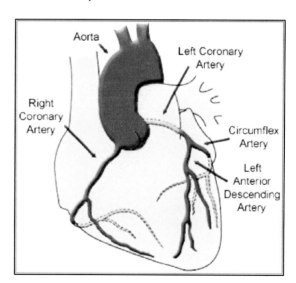

Coronary Anatomy

In general, disease in the coronary arteries affects the walls as follows:

- **Left anterior descending artery disease** affects the:
  - anterior
  - septal
  - anterior free wall
  - anterior left ventricle apex

Depending on **diagonal branches**, the lateral wall may also be affected.

- If the **left anterior descending artery wraps around the apex**, then the following walls are affected:
  - apical segments
  - inferior and posterolateral walls

Remember, the location of the lesion in this artery also determines which areas are affected.

- Disease in the **circumflex artery** can affect the:
  - Lateral wall
  - Inferolateral LV wall

Conventional or stress echocardiography may be especially useful for patients with circumflex disease since this region may not be well visualized in single-plane,
right anterior oblique left ventriculograms. Disease in this area is often "silent" on the electrocardiogram.

- Disease of the **posterior descending artery** may cause motion abnormalities of the:
  - Inferior free wall
  - Inferior interventricular
  - septum
  - Inferolateral left ventricle segments
  - If the apex is supplied by the posterior descending artery it may be affected extensively.

Branches of the three main vessels can cause more discrete motion abnormalities. **Proximal right coronary artery disease** may cause problems in the right ventricular free wall and diagonal branch disease may affect the inferior wall. The distal right coronary artery affects the inferior wall of the left ventricle.

The heart walls are divided to determine the regions affected by disease. The breakdown of the cardiac walls was covered in chapter one.

Left ventricular function and regional ventricular function can be assessed. The ejection fraction gives important clinical information in patients with coronary artery disease. 2-D evaluation works best when multiple tomographic planes are employed and the endocardium is well defined. Several methods for evaluating 2-D left ventricular function can be used. Tracing and measuring the left ventricle and the endocardium in multiple tomographic planes during systole and diastole is the primary component of several of these methods.

When regional wall motion abnormalities are present, Simpson's rule is often a good measurement of left ventricular function. This is also referred to as the Method of Discs **(MOD)** or summation of discs. The ventricle is measured from the base to apex in a series of discs. The modified Simpson's rule approximation uses three parallel slices of the ventricle to obtain the volume.

Wall motion scoring should be performed in several tomographic planes. The walls are graded on a scale of one to five based on the function.

1 **Normal**
2 **Hypokinesia**
3 **Akinesis**
4 **Dyskinesis**
5 **Aneurysm**

The overall wall **motion score index** is calculated by the equation:

WMSI =
sum of individual segment scores
# of segments visualized

A perfusion defect greater than 20% should be suspected when the WMSI is greater than 1.7.

Echocardiography has evolved over the years and is an important diagnostic tool used in the determination and management of patients with a suspected acute myocardial infarction.

Echocardiography can help to exclude an acute myocardial infarction on those patients that present with chest pain, but have non-diagnostic EKG's. When it is determined that an acute event has occurred, echocardiography can help to determine the size of the infarction and the benefits of reperfusion therapy. Echocardiography can also help in the determination of complications associated with infarction, the viability of the myocardium, and the potential associated with infarction, and the potential risks to the patient.

When 2-D imaging is performed on a patient with ischemia or myocardial infarction, several factors should be considered:

- A patient at rest with no previous myocardial infarction or angina at the time of the echocardiogram should have normal wall motion.
- If a patient is having chest pain during an echocardiogram, the myocardium may be hypokinetic, dyskinetic, or akinetic.
- Echocardiography cannot distinguish acute myocardial infarction from ischemia, only the presence of the motion abnormality.
- A patient with normal wall motion and pain, typically has a low probability of an acute myocardial infarction.

- A patient having an acute myocardial infarction presents with a wall motion abnormality, possible abnormal EKG findings, and elevated serum cardiac enzymes, but not always. The region of the abnormality may be normal in thickness and may even be somewhat thickened due to edema, but both diastolic and systolic function is abnormal.

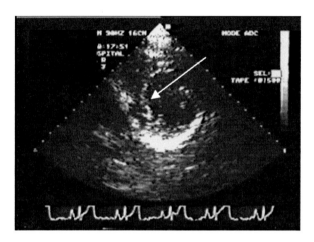

Short Axis View Acute MI

With a **transmural infarction** that involves 50% or more of the wall thickness, the region will begin to thin, increase in echogenicity, and become akinetic approximately 4-6 weeks after the initial event. A **non-transmural infarction** of less than 50% typically results in walls that are less thinned and hypokinetic.

A chronic infarct appears as a region with a motion abnormality, thinned wall, and often increased in echogenicity due to scarring. In both chronic and acute infarction, adjacent or opposite walls may have compensatory hyperkinesis. When a patient having a prior myocardial infarction presents with new

195

chest pain, it may be difficult to detect the area of the new infarction if it is located adjacent to the old one.

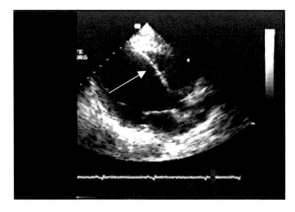

Chronic IVS Infarction

When an **inferior wall myocardial infarction** is detected, the right ventricle should be evaluated since up to 40% involve the right ventricle. The right ventricle may be dilated, the free wall hypokinetic, arrhythmia's and hypotension may be present, and tricuspid regurgitation can result.

A patient with an **anterior myocardial infarction** may have as much as 40% ischemia of left ventricular myocardium. Patient outcome and survival may be correlated with the severity of the left ventricular dysfunction.

M-mode findings seen with a chronic infarction may show thinning of the wall, abnormal wall motion, and increased echogenicity.

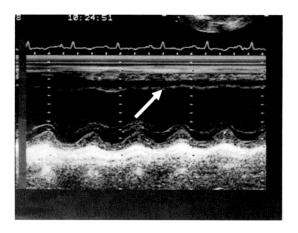

M-Mode of Chronic IVS Infarction

New infarcts may have normal or thick walls, but a motion abnormality will be present. Adjacent or opposing walls may be hyperkinetic if an abnormality is present. The EPSS may be increased due to the left ventricular dysfunction and the ejection fraction may be abnormal, if systolic dysfunction is extensive.

The Doppler exam in an acute infarction shows diastolic dysfunction with a low E to A velocity ratio on the inflow. If reperfusion is successful, this may return to normal. If the infarct is large and reperfusion does not occur, the E velocity increases due to increased left ventricular end diastolic pressures

ASSOCIATED FINDINGS

There are several complications associated with a myocardial infarction. Any time there is a wall motion abnormality and stasis of flow, mural thrombus can occur. 17-20% of patients develop thrombus, but only 2-12% have systemic emboli. The incidence of thrombus is increased when any or all of the following are present:

- Overall left ventricular function is decreased
- Aneurysm
- Wall motion abnormality
- Spontaneous contrast in the left ventricle

Spontaneous contrast is caused by a low output state resulting in the clumping of red blood cells to the point of being echo reflective. Very rarely do thrombi occur in the absence of wall motion abnormalities. This can occur in patients with hypereosinophilic syndrome. A patient with this condition may develop thrombus in the left ventricle apex and mitral valve area.

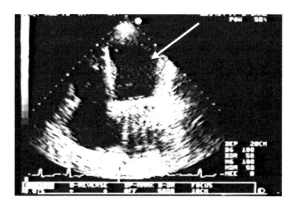

Spontaneous Contrast

Thrombus often occurs six days or so post myocardial infarction. Thrombus often may be difficult to identify due to its decreased or isoechoic echotexture. The endocardial surface should be carefully examined for unusual areas of increased echogenicity or abnormal thickening. Thrombi may bulge into the left ventricle or can be laminated against the walls.

Prominent apical trabeculations or false tendons may be confused for thrombus. Apical thrombus is common. A thrombus is more commonly seen in patients with an anterior myocardial infarction. Detection of an apical thrombus may be difficult to detect due to its location in the near field and associated artifacts. Use of a higher frequency transducer, adjustment of the focal zones, injection of contrast agents, and multiple imaging planes may help to offset these problems.

Aneurysms may occur after a myocardial infarction. Apical aneurysms are the most common, however infero-basal aneurysms are possible. A left ventricular aneurysm presents as a dyskinetic area having a diastolic contour abnormality, and thinned walls. These are also called true aneurysms. Approximately 15-25% of patients with an acute myocardial infarction may develop a left ventricular true aneurysm. Clot may be present within an aneurysm. This type of an aneurysm needs to be differentiated from a Takotsubo Cardiomyopathy due to its apical ballooning. The neck diameter of a true aneurysm is larger than that of a pseudoaneurysm.

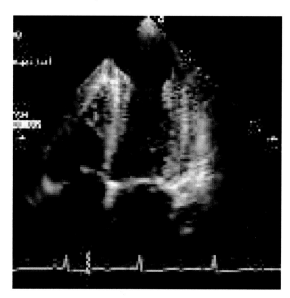

True Apical Aneurysm

Play Video 7A: Akinetic apex with apical clot

Play Video 7B: LV apical aneurysm with spontaneous contrast

Pseudoaneurysm is another complication that may occur after a myocardial infarction. A pseudo aneurysm is a ventricular free wall rupture of the myocardium which is contained by the pericardium. A pseudoaneurysm is a surgical emergency and needs to be differentiated from a true aneurysm. A pseudoaneurysm is a rare complication that occurs less than 1% of cases, but are considered a surgical emergency since up to 30% rupture.

If rupture occurs, pericardial effusion is typically present with the possibility of tamponade. Occasionally, patients have containment of the rupture due to thrombus or adhesions.

On the 2-D exam a pseudoaneurysm has a narrow neck at the rupture site and the transition from the normal myocardium to the aneurysm is abrupt. The ratio of the neck diameter to the aneurysm is less than 0.5 cm. There is usually flow in and out of the pseudoaneurysm that can typically be detected with color flow imaging. If present, clot formation within the pseudoaneurysm can be observed using the parasternal long axis, apical two, three, and four chamber views of the heart.

The most common locations for a pseudoaneurysm is at the posterior and lateral walls of the LV.

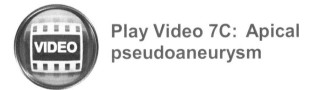

Play Video 7C: Apical pseudoaneurysm

Valvular dysfunction, especially involving the mitral valve, may occur as a complication of myocardial infarction. Often times after the infarction, a patient may present with a new murmur, the mitral valve is commonly the source. Mitral valve dysfunction is typically due to papillary muscle dysfunction, abnormal wall motion of the segment under the papillary muscle, or papillary muscle rupture. When an inferior myocardial infarction occurs, mitral regurgitation most likely results from papillary muscle dysfunction. With an anterior myocardial infarction, the cause of mitral regurgitation is often due to dilatation of the left ventricle and valve annulus. Mitral regurgitation results in up to 60% of patients with an anterior myocardial infarction.

Papillary muscle rupture is usually a complication associated with an inferior wall myocardial infarction. The posterior medial papillary muscle is most commonly affected. The mitral leaflet becomes flail resulting in moderate to severe acute mitral regurgitation.

Pericardial effusion may be a finding in post infarction patients. This is called Dressler's syndrome and usually occurs 6-10 days after the infarction. Effusions are usually small to moderate and rarely results in tamponade.

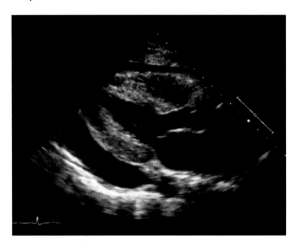

Dressler's Syndrome – Pericardial effusion post MI

Ventricular septal defects may occur and are usually a result of small infarcts that cause necrosis and rupture of a focal area. Shunts are high velocity, left to right, and the prognosis is poor.

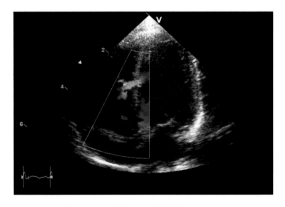

Muscular VSD on A4C view

Ischemic cardiomyopathy may occur in patients with multi-vessel disease and previous infarcts. This is caused by severe coronary insufficiency and subsequent progressive heart failure, rather than episodes of angina and infarction.

Play Video 7D:
Dilated cardiomyopathy

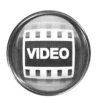

Play Video 7E:
PLAX Ruptured IVS Post MI

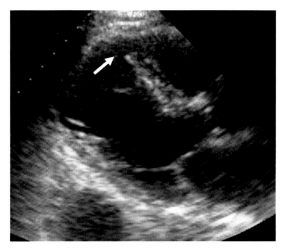

Right Ventricular Involvement

Play Video 7F:
Apical Long Ruptured IVS Post MI

It is not uncommon for the right heart to be involved in an acute myocardial infarction, but typically it is not hemodynamically significant. Hemo- dynamically significant right ventricular involvement is typically associated with an inferior wall myocardial infarction.

Patients' presenting with hypoxemia post inferior wall myocardial infarction should be evaluated for a right ventricular infarction and possible right-to-left shunt through a patent foramen ovale.

ECHO INDICATIONS OF RIGHT VENTRICULAR MYOCARDIAL INFARCTION

- Dilated right ventricle
- Hypokinetic or akinetic right ventricle
- Dilated right atrium
- Significant tricuspid regurgitation
- Possible right-to-left shunt if a patent foramen ovale is present

Initially, myocardial ischemia affects the diastolic function of the left ventricle due to myocardial relaxation that is both prolonged and delayed. The effect of this diastolic dysfunction results in a prolonged isovolumetric relaxation time, lower transmitral pressure gradient during mitral valve opening, and consequently a decrease of the early rapid filling of the left ventricle. The E velocity deceleration becomes prolonged due to the slow relaxation. The left atrium does not completely empty which causes an increased left atrial contraction, and therefore an increased A velocity.

Typical Mitral Flow Patterns Associated with Relaxation Abnormalities

- Decreased E velocity
- Increased deceleration time of E velocity
- Increased A velocity
- Decreased E to A ratio

ABNORMAL MYOCARDIAL RELAXATION

When a patient experiences a myocardial infarction, there can be a variety of effects on the mitral flow velocity pattern depending upon several possible events.

Factors Affecting Mitral Flow Velocity After a Myocardial Infarction

- Left atrial pressure
- Heart rate
- Loading conditions

- Relaxation abnormalities
- Ventricular compliance
- Pericardial compliance
- Atrial fibrillation

Left atrial pressure may be one of the most intense factors affecting the diastolic filling pattern. When the left atrial pressure is increased, the diastolic filling pattern is restrictive. Patients having a restrictive diastolic filling pattern after an acute myocardial infarction are at a greater risk of developing heart failure.

Restrictive Diastolic Filling Patterns

- Increased E velocity
- Decreased A velocity
- Decreased deceleration time
- Increased E to A ratio

NORMAL LVF

Left ventricular function is one of the most important objectives for performing an echocardiogram. Systolic left ventricular function plays a prime role in every aspect of the exam whether it is the focus of that exam or not. Normal systole occurs from mitral valve closure to aortic valve closure or when left ventricular diastolic pressure exceeds left atrial pressure. When systole occurs, the left ventricle contracts. The contractility of the left ventricle can be affected by preload and afterload.

Diastole is the interval from the aortic valve closure to the mitral valve closure and is divided into four phases:

Four Phases of Diastole

1. Isovolumetric relaxation
2. Early rapid diastolic filling phase
3. Diastasis
4. Late diastolic filling due to atrial contraction

The left ventricle pressure falls quickly during isovolumetric relaxation after the aortic valve closes. When the pressure in the left ventricle decreases below the left atrial pressure, the mitral valve opens. Diastasis is the period of time when the flow between the left atrium and left ventricle equalizes, followed by the left atrial contraction. Left atrial contraction contributes approximately 20-30% of the blood towards left ventricular filling.

Diastolic Function

Diastolic function can be assessed through the diastolic filling patterns. Myocardial compliance and relaxation change with age and with almost all types of cardiac disease. As aging occurs, the rate of left ventricular elastic recoil and myocardial relaxation decreases. When this occurs, the left ventricular pressure decreases resulting in slower filling. The effects of aging on diastolic function are indicated by a longer isovolumetric relaxation time and a lower E velocity. It is not abnormal to find an E/A ratio < 1.0 in patients over age 70.

Normal Diastolic Filling/No Anatomic Abnormalities

Deceleration Time 160-240 msec (may be lower in young patients)
Isovolumetric relaxation time 70-90 msec
E/A ratio 1-2
Mitral A duration ≥ PVa duration
PVs2 ≥ PVd (can be reversed in young patients)

Source: The Echo Manual (Oh et al.)

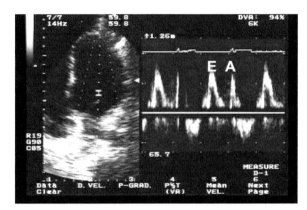

Normal LV Inflow Pattern

Two types of patterns can be found with left ventricular diastolic dysfunction: patterns associated with impaired myocardial relaxation and patterns associated with restrictive filling or decreased compliance.

COMMON CAUSES OF IMPAIRED MYOCARDIAL RELAXATION

- Left ventricular hypertrophy
- Myocardial Ischemia or Infarction
- Hypertrophic Cardiomyopathy
- Age

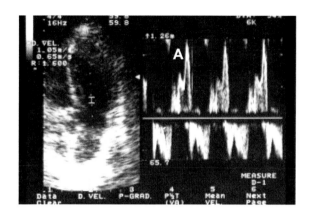

Doppler Flow Pattern Associated with Impaired Myocardial Relaxation

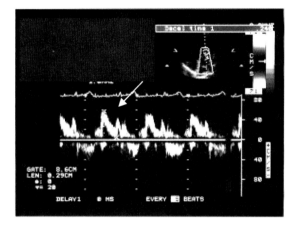

Normal LV Inflow Pattern

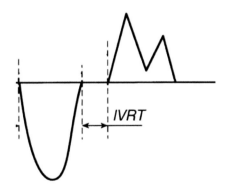

Isovolumetric Relaxation Time Measurement (Measured from AV closure to MV opening)

201

Impaired Relaxation Diastolic Filling

Deceleration Time   > 200msec
Isovolumetric Relaxation Time > 90msec
E/A < 1.0
PVs2 > PVd
Mitral A duration ≥ or < PVa duration (depends on Left Ventricular End Diastolic Pressures)

Source: The Echo Manual (Oh et al.)

Restrictive filling or decreased compliance can be found in a number of cardiac abnormalities. This physiology occurs when left ventricular compliance is decreased and left atrial pressure is increased. The increase in the left atrial pressure causes the mitral valve to open sooner, consequently decreasing isovolumetric relaxation time and increasing the E velocity.

CAUSES OF RESTRICTIVE FILLING

- Severe Coronary Artery Disease
- Acute, severe aortic regurgitation
- Congestive Heart Failure (decompensated)
- Constrictive Pericarditis
- Restrictive Cardiomyopathy

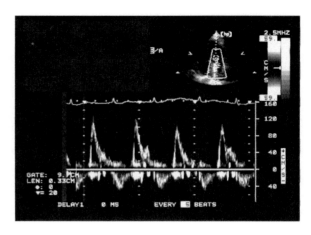

Doppler Flow Pattern Associated with Restrictive Filling (Decreased Compliance)

Restrictive Diastolic Filling

Deceleration Time < 160msec
Isovolumic Relaxation Time < 70msec
E/A ratio > 1.5
PVs2 << PVd
Mitral A duration < PVa duration
PVa velocity increased (≥ 35cm/sec, but not always.

Source: The Echo Manual (Oh et al.)

Pseudo normalization of the diastolic filling patterns occurs when diastolic dysfunction worsens and changes from impaired relaxation to restrictive filling. A period of transition results in what appears to be normal diastolic filling patterns. Pseudo normalization is caused from left atrial pressures that are moderately increased and that are imposed over a relaxation abnormality.

VENTRICULAR FUNCTION QUIZ

1. When a wall motion abnormality lasts for 24-72 hours, but has not had irreversible damage, it is referred to as:
   a. hibernating
   b. necrotic
   c. stunned
   d. spastic

2. When tissue is abnormal at rest, but functions with reperfusion through exercise or medication, it is referred to as:
   a. hibernating
   b. stunned
   c. shocked
   d. necrotic

3. When the heart wall has absent inward wall motion and lacks systolic thickening, it is said to be:
   a. Hypokinetic
   b. hyperkinetic
   c. akinetic
   d. dyskinetic

4. When a segment of the heart wall bulges in systole and appears thinned and moves paradoxically as compared with the surrounding myocardium, it is:
   a. akinetic
   b. dyskinetic
   c. hypokinetic
   d. hyperkinetic

5. Approximately ___% of patients have left dominant coronary artery circulation.
   a. 20%
   b. 40%
   c. 60%
   d. 80%

6. Disease in the left anterior descending artery affects all of the following EXCEPT:
   a. anterior LV apex
   b. right ventricle free wall
   c. septum
   d. anterior wall

7. Echocardiography is often helpful in patients with circumflex disease because
   a. this region is often "silent" on the EKG
   b. this region is not well visualized in a single plane right anterior oblique left ventriculogram
   c. most people have left dominant coronary artery circulation
   d. all of the above
   e. a & b only

8. The two walls seen in the apical two chamber view are the:
   a. inferior wall
   b. anterior wall
   c. inferolateral wall
   d. lateral wall
   e. a and b
   f. c and d

9. The MOD or summation of discs is also known as:
   a. Bernoulli equation
   b. Bullet rule
   c. Modified Simpson's rule
   d. Teicholtz equation

10. Which of the following is an ultrasound characteristic of acute myocardial infarction?
    a. normal or thickened walls of the affected area
    b. systolic dysfunction of the affected area
    c. diastolic dysfunction of the affected area
    d. all of the above

11. Which of the following is NOT a typical 2-D finding in the region of a chronic infarction?
    a. thin wall
    b. increased echogenicity of the affected wall or region
    c. decreased echogenicity of the affected wall or region
    d. abnormal wall motion

12. The right ventricle may be involved up to 40% of the time in patients with infarctions of the:
    a. anterior wall
    b. inferolateral wall
    c. inferior wall
    d. anterolateral wall

13. The incidence of left ventricular thrombus increases when all of the following are present except:
    a. overall left ventricular function is decreased
    b. aneurysm
    c. pericardial effusion
    d. spontaneous contrast

14. Thrombus usually occurs approximately the _____day after a myocardial infarction.
    a. Second
    b. Fourth
    c. Sixth
    d. Eighth

15. Which of the following is NOT considered a phase of diastole?
    a. early or rapid filling
    b. diastasis
    c. atrial contraction
    d. isovolumetric contraction time

16. Which of the following is NOT a confusing condition for LV thrombus?
    a. moderator band
    b. false tendon
    c. prominent apical trabeculations
    d. abnormally located papillary muscle

17. The most common location for an aneurysm to occur is the:
    a. inferobasal wall b. LV apex
    c. interventricular septum
    d. all walls can be equally affected

18. In determining a pseudoaneurysm from a true aneurysm, the ratio of the neck diameter to the aneurysm is:
    a. > 1.0 cm
    b. < 1.0 cm
    c. < 1.5 cm
    d. < 0.5 cm

19. When a patient presents with a new murmur after a myocardial infarction, the source is often the:
    a. aortic valve
    b. tricuspid valve
    c. pulmonic valve
    d. mitral valve

20. Mitral regurgitation associated with papillary muscle dysfunction is the result of:
    a. an inferior wall myocardial infarction
    b. an anterior wall myocardial infarction
    c. a posterior wall myocardial infarction
    d. an apical infarction

21. A pericardial effusion occurring 6-10 days after a myocardial infarction is called:
    a. Marfan's syndrome
    b. Barlow's syndrome
    c. Dressler's syndrome
    d. Dressback's syndrome

22. Dilatation of the mitral valve annulus with subsequent mitral regurgitation is usually a result of:
   a. an inferior wall myocardial infarction
   b. an anterior wall myocardial infarction
   c. a inferolateral wall myocardial infarction
   d. an apical infarction

23. The period of time when flow between the left atrium and left ventricle equalizes is:
   a. isovolumetric relaxation
   b. diastasis
   c. late diastolic filling
   d. early rapid diastolic filling

24. The image below indicates a (an)
   a. pseudoaneurysm
   b. apical aneurysm
   c. apical thrombus
   d. ruptured interventricular septum

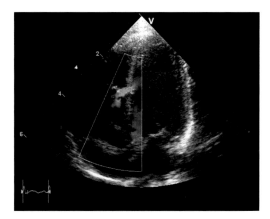

25. The Doppler tracing below demonstrates what type of flow pattern?
   a. impaired relaxation
   b. restrictive filling
   c. normal inflow
   d. normal outflow

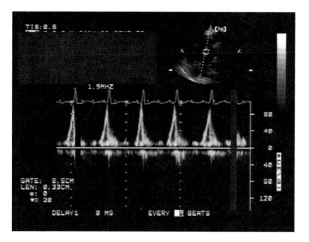

26. Some ventricular septal defects occur due to _____myocardial infarction and create a _____ to _____shunt.
   a. large; right to left
   b. small; right to left
   c. large; left to right
   d. small; left to right

27. Diagnose the following 2D image in a patient post myocardial infarction:
   a. Mitral stenosis
   b. Papillary rupture
   c. True Aneurysm
   d. Dressler's syndrome

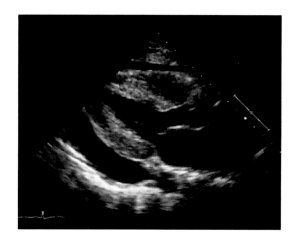

28. Diagnose the following complication due to a myocardial infarction:
    a. True aneurysm
    b. Dressler's syndrome
    c. Ventricular septal defect
    d. Papillary muscle dysfunction

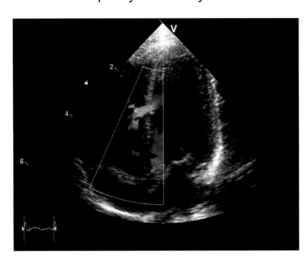

30. What component of echo is most helpful in the diagnosis of a pseudoaneurysm:

    a. 2D imaging
    b. M-mode
    c. Color flow imaging
    d. Continuous wave Doppler

29. The following color abnormality is most likely due to a:
    a. Pericardial effusion
    b. True Aneurysm
    c. Mitral valve prolapse
    d. Papillary muscle dysfunction

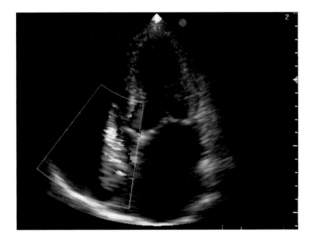

GULFCOAST
ULTRASOUND
INSTITUTE INC

Section 8:

Cardiac Tumors

Section 8: CARDIAC TUMORS

Objectives

Upon completion of this module you should be able to:

- Differentiate primary and secondary cardiac tumors

- Recognize the complications associated with cardiac tumors

- Identify the pericardial involvement of cardiac tumors

- Apply echocardiography methods to differentiate other masses and artifacts from cardiac tumors

Cardiac Tumors

BENIGN TUMORS

Approximately 75% of primary cardiac tumors are benign. As with most tumors, this determination is made pathologically. The heart can be affected by tumors through the invasion of the myocardium, epicardium, or pericardium, due to the production of substances that are biologically active, and from the toxic effects that treatment for various cancers can have on the heart.

__Myxomas__ comprise approximately 27% of the primary cardiac tumors. Myxomas are rare in children, but are three times more common in women with a possible familial occurrence. Approximately 75% of myxomas occur in the left atrium and tend to be single. Typically, myxomas arise from the fossa ovalis of the interatrial septum. They can also occur in the right atrium, left ventricle, and right ventricle. Approximately 5% of patients with myxomas have multiple lesions.

The clinical presentation may include fever and malaise. Obstructive symptoms similar to those with mitral stenosis may occur if the tumor obstructs left atrial flow. Emboli are also possible. Symptoms associated with tumor obstruction may include: seizures, syncope, coma, shock, acute pulmonary edema, cyanosis, gangrene of the nose and toes, and episodes of bizarre behavior. Positional changes may affect symptoms.

The 2-D exam typically demonstrates the myxoma that can be variable in size, shape, and echogenicity. A myxoma can completely fill the atria and prolapse into the ventricle. On auscultation this event is referred to as a tumor "plop". The mass may be irregular with a non-homogeneous texture. Calcifications may be seen within the mass. Multiple views are helpful in locating the myxoma and its point of

attachment. Myxomas may reoccur after surgical excision and often grow more rapidly the second time.

On the Doppler exam the degree of tumor obstruction may be determined by a pressure half- time measurement of the mitral valve flow.

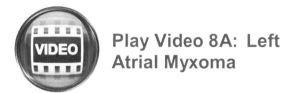

Play Video 8A: Left Atrial Myxoma

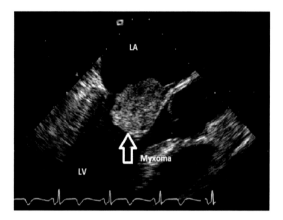

Left Atrial Myxoma on TEE

Papillary fibroelastomas are benign cardiac tumors that usually occur in valve tissue. The mitral valve is most often affected, but they can occur on the aortic valve. These tumors are histologically similar to Lambl's excrescence's seen in the elderly as a normal finding. They usually attach on the left ventricle side of the mitral valve and the aortic side of the aortic valve. They often have the appearance of a vegetation, except for their location. These tumors usually have no clinical importance.

__Rhabdomyomas__ are tumors that usually attach to areas of the septum. They are the most common cardiac tumor seen in children and are often associated with tuberous sclerosis. Rhabdomyomas are typically egg-shaped, multiple and highly invasive.

211

Tuberous sclerosis is a syndrome manifested by convulsive seizures, progressive mental disorders, adenoma sebacum, and benign tumors of the kidneys, heart and brain.

Hemangiomas may be seen in the adult and are benign tumors composed of multiple small blood vessels.

Mesotheliomas are tumors that occur on the AV node and can cause complete heart block, Stokes-Adams syncope, and sudden death. These tumors are small, slow growing, cystic tumors. This tumor almost always occurs in adults and predominantly in women.

Lipomatous hypertrophy of the interatrial septum may appear like a cardiac mass. It usually involves the fatty portion of the superior and inferior interatrial septum resulting in a dumbbell-shaped septum.

MALIGNANT TUMORS

Primary malignant tumors are rare and account for approximately 20% of cardiac tumors. They are almost exclusively sarcomas and can occur in all age groups with no gender distinction.

Clinically, there may be cardiac failure, cardiomegaly, hemopericardium, chest pain, and cardiac rhythm disturbances. Secondary cardiac tumors are 20-40 times more common than primary tumors.

Metastasis to the pericardium occurs more frequently than to the myocardium. The most common metastatic tumors arise from the breast and lungs, occurring in approximately 1/3 of cases. Malignant tumors that may involve the myocardium of the heart are typically lymphomas or melanomas. Malignant melanoma may involve the myocardium in greater than 50% of cases, but is basically uncommon.

Metastatic tumors reach the heart via embolic hematogenous spread, lymphatic spread, or direct invasion. Carcinoma of the bronchus and breast frequently spread via the lymphatics. Lymphomas related to AIDS frequently involve the heart extensively.

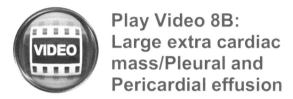

Play Video 8B: Large extra cardiac mass/Pleural and Pericardial effusion

Pericardial Involvement

Approximately 75% of metastatic cardiac disease affects the pericardium and epicardium, typically causing a pericardial effusion. Metastatic involvement with a pericardial effusion can be determined by evaluating the pericardial fluid or possible pericardial biopsy. Patients with known cancer and pericardial effusion may have radiation pericarditis or idiopathic pericarditis, a common occurrence in cancer patients. The prognosis for a patient with a malignant pericardial effusion is poor. The estimated 1-year survival rate is less than 50%.

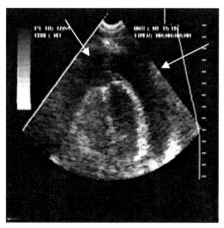

Malignant Pericardial Effusion

Renal cell carcinoma, Wilm's tumors (common in children), and uterine tumors can metastasize to the heart via extension through the inferior vena cava.

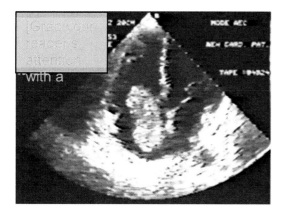

Renal Cell Carcinoma Extending into Heart via the **IVC**

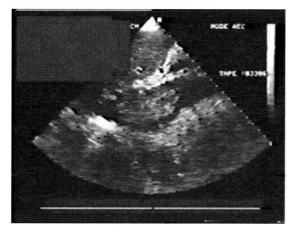

Renal Cell Carcinoma Extension into the Right Side of Heart

Tumors can indirectly affect the heart such as **carcinoid heart disease**. This typically involves the right side of the heart and produces a biologically active material that affects the cardiac valves and endocardium. Thickening, stiffness, and retraction of the pulmonic and tricuspid valves occurs resulting in valves that are "stuck half way open".

Consequently, valvular regurgitation and stenosis may result from carcinoid heart disease. While carcinoid heart disease is uncommon, half of those who have carcinoid involvement die from heart failure as a result of severe tricuspid regurgitation or extension of the disease to the left heart through a patent foramen ovale.

Tumors that may affect the heart due to extra- cardiac compression are variable. Hematomas, thyomas, cysts of the mediastinum, and teratomas may be responsible. Teratomas usually arise near the roots of the great vessels and are usually multicystic, firm, and well-encapsulated in adults.

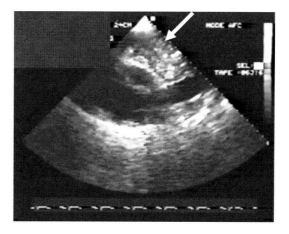

Mediastinal Mass Compressing Heart

Masses in the mediastinum may be large enough to compress the heart. Pancreatic cysts, abdominal masses, and diaphragmatic hernias may cause extra- cardiac compression.

Tumors of the pleura, associated with pleural effusions may also cause cardiac compression.

DIFFERENTIATION FROM OTHER MASSES OR ARTIFACTS

Differential findings of masses in the heart are variable. **Cardiac thrombus** is more commonly seen on the left side, however right sided thrombus can occur as well as a thrombus in-transit. Thrombus that is seen in the left ventricle usually occurs in regions where there is stasis of blood. These areas include: wall motion abnormalities, aneurysm, pseudoaneurysm, and patients with dilated cardiomyopathies.

Even when thrombus is not seen in patients with these conditions, there is a high possibility for thrombus when the ejection fraction is less than 20%. The identification of left ventricular thrombus requires multiple views, as well as careful adjustment of gain controls and possibly a higher frequency transducer to obtain optimum detail.

Thrombus can have a similar appearance as the heart wall. Fresh thrombus may be hypoechoic to anechoic while older thrombus may be somewhat increased in echogenicity.

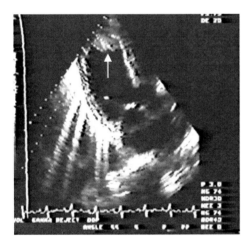

Left Ventricular Thrombus

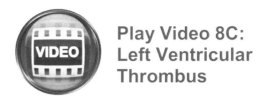

Play Video 8C: Left Ventricular Thrombus

Trabeculations, false tendons, abnormally located papillary muscles, and redundant chordae may result in false positive findings.

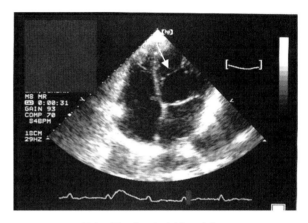

False Tendon Left Ventricle

Left atrial clots tend to be more difficult to visualize on the transthoracic exam due to location of the atrium. Left atrial clots are usually associated with an enlarged left atrium, mitral valve disease, and atrial fibrillation. Patients with mitral regurgitation may have a slightly decreased chance for clot due to the movement of blood by the regurgitant jet.

Clot in the left atrium is difficult to find not only due to the location of the left atrium, but because left atrial thrombus commonly occurs in the left atrial appendage. This region may be seen from a parasternal short axis view or an apical two chamber view with a slight superior angulation. A negative finding for a left atrial clot does not exclude the possibility nor does a positive finding rule one in. Transthoracic echocardiography is usually less than adequate when a left atrial clot is suspected.

Transesophageal echocardiography is more accurate for the detection of left atrial clot. Clots may be missed in the heart if they are small. Typically, clots need to be greater than 6mm to be detected.

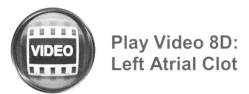

Play Video 8D:
Left Atrial Clot

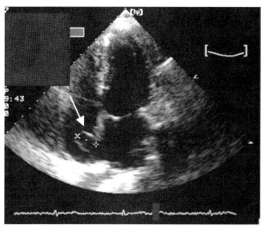

Interatrial Septal Aneurysm Apical Four Chamber View

Aneurysms of the interatrial septum, cor triatriatum, dilated coronary sinus, anomalous pulmonary venous return, and lipomatous hypertrophy of the interatrial septum can also cause an unusual appearance to the atria.

An aneurysm of the interatrial septum can be detected when the interatrial septum bulges greater than 15mm from the septal plane and there is no elevation of right or left atrial pressures. An aneurysm of the interatrial septum is associated in 90% of cases with fenestration, an opening closed by a membrane. Interatrial septal aneurysms occur in the region of the fossa ovalis. There is some association between these aneurysms and increased risk of systemic embolic events and atrial arrhythmias.

Cor triatriatum is a perforated muscular membrane that separates the atrium into upper and lower chambers. The membrane is usually above the atrial appendage, but below the pulmonary veins.

Anomalous pulmonary venous return is an abnormal connection of the pulmonary veins. There are two types, complete and partial depending on venous connections.

Lipomatous hypertrophy of the interatrial septum may appear like a cardiac mass. It usually involves the inferior and superior portions of the interatrial septum and does not affect the fossa ovalis.

Right heart thrombus is uncommon, but may be seen in patients with severe right ventricular dilatation and dysfunction. Venous thrombus can embolize to the heart and is a more common cause of right sided thrombus. Catheters and pacer wires may be a source of right atrial thrombus. These may also be a source of a false positive finding sometimes giving an abnormal, but indistinguishable appearance in the heart chambers. The moderator band in the right ventricle, trabeculations, abnormally located papillary muscles and redundant chordae may also be confused for clots or masses. Occasionally the Eustachian valve can be seen and confused for a right atrial mass.

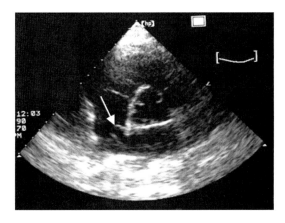

Interatrial Septal Aneurysm Parasternal Short Axis View

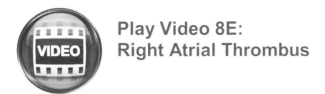

Play Video 8E:
Right Atrial Thrombus

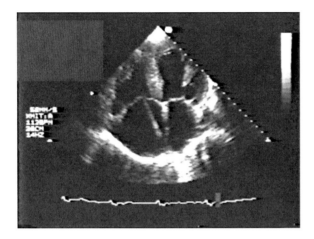

Pacemaker Wire Right Heart

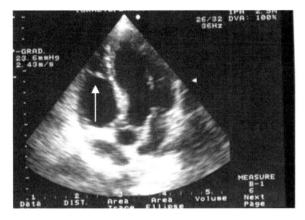

Moderator Band Right Ventricle

A **Chiari network** is a fibrous-appearing structure found in the right atrium. A Chiari's network is a prominent inferior vena cava valve that extends into the coronary sinus and/or the crista terminalis.

CARDIAC TUMORS QUIZ

1. The most common benign primary cardiac tumor is the:
   a. rhabdomyoma
   b. sarcoma
   c. myxoma
   d. papilloma

2. Approximately what percent of cardiac tumors are benign?
   a. 20%
   b. 27%
   c. 75%
   d. 90%

3. The most common site for a myxoma is:
   a. right atrium
   b. left atrium
   c. left ventricle
   d. right ventricle

4. Which valve is most often affected by papillary fibroelastomas?
   a. mitral valve
   b. aortic valve
   c. tricuspid valve
   d. pulmonic valve

5. Which type of tumor is associated with tuberous sclerosis?
   a. sarcomas
   b. myxomas
   c. teratomas
   d. rhabdomyomas

6. What tumor occurs on the AV node?
   a. hemangioma
   b. teratomas
   c. mesotheliomas
   d. lymphomas

7. The most common metastatic tumors are from the:
   a. lung
   b. ovary
   c. breast
   d. uterus
   e. b and c
   f. a and c

8. Malignant tumors that may involve the myocardium are usually:
   a. hemangiomas
   b. lymphoma
   c. melanoma
   d. myxoma
   e. a & d
   f. b & c

9. Carcinoid heart disease usually involves the right heart and produces biologically active material that affects the cardiac valves and the _____.
   a. endocardium
   b. myocardium
   c. epicardium
   d. unicardium

10. Which of the following tumors invade the heart via extension through the IVC?
    a. renal cell carcinoma
    b. rhabdomyoma
    c. Wilm's tumor
    d. teratoma
    e. a and c
    f. b and c

11. Lipomatous hypertrophy may look like a mass and commonly involves the:
    a. interventricular septum
    b. interatrial septum
    c. apex
    d. left ventricle

12. A fibrous appearing structure found in the right atrium may be a:
    a. right coronary artery
    b. Chiari's network
    c. moderator band
    d. coronary sinus

217

13. Which of the following is NOT a probable source of right atrial thrombus?
    a. catheters
    b. pacer wires
    c. venous thrombus
    d. arterial thrombus   .

14. An aneurysm of the interatrial septum is considered when septal bulging is greater than _____ from the septal plane.
    a. 10 mm
    b. 15 mm
    c. 5 mm
    d. 3 mm

15. In order for clots to be detected in the left atrium, the clots usually need to be greater than _____mm.
    a. 3
    b. 4
    c. 5
    d. 6

16. Diagnose the following image:
    a. Lipomatous hypertrophy
    b. Papilloma
    c. Eustachian valve
    d. Myxoma

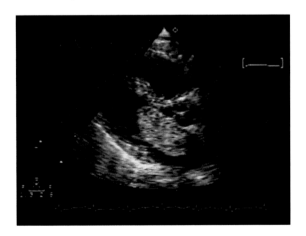

17. The most common benign valvular tumor is known as:
    a. Myxoma
    b. Angiosarcoma
    c. Papillary fibroelastoma
    d. Lipoma

18. The most common benign cardiac tumor found in children is known as a:
    a. Myxoma
    b. Rhabdomyoma
    c. Angiosarcoma
    d. Papillary fibroelastoma

19. The most common malignant tumor is called:
    a. Sarcoma
    b. Myxoma
    c. Rhabdomyoma
    d. Lipoma

20. Select three benign cardiac tumors:
    Lipoma
    Angiosarcoma
    Fibroma
    Teratoma
    Rhabdomyosarcoma
    Lymphoma
    Myxosarcoma

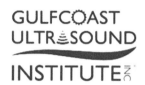

Section 9:

Miscellaneous

Section 9: MISCELLANEOUS

Objectives

Upon completion of this module you should be able to:

- Identify various arrhythmias and conduction disturbances as they relate to the echocardiogram

- State the effect of arrhythmias and conduction disturbances on the cardiac valves

- Apply the parameters of left ventricular function

- Identify the findings associated with right side volume overload

- Relate the effects of arrhythmias and conduction disturbances to the Doppler flow velocity waveforms

- Identify various other cardiac diagnostic examinations

- Demonstrate knowledge of basic cardiovascular medications

MISCELLANEOUS

ARRHYTHMIAS AND CONDUCTION DISTURBANCES

Even though the echocardiogram evaluates mechanical function of the heart, electrical disturbances may affect and alter mechanical function and appearance of the structures on the exam. This may be especially evident on the M-mode and tissue Doppler exams where the faster sampling rates have the ability to detect subtle and rapid motion changes.

Patients with a **left bundle branch block** usually have changes in the motion of the interventricular septum. This is noted by a quick, early, negative motion in systole that is followed by a gradual anterior displacement of the interventricular septum lasting throughout ventricular ejection. The primary feature on the echocardiogram of a left bundle branch block is the downward movement of the interventricular septum occurring at the start of electrical depolarization. In addition, with tissue Doppler imaging, the septal-to-posterior-wall delay may be measured.

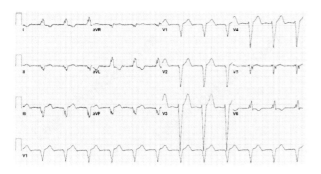

12-Lead ECG of LBBB

Patient's with **Wolff-Parkinson-White syndrome** also have certain characteristic findings. This is an abnormality of the conduction rhythm that manifests as supraventricular tachycardia. Diagnosis is made on the EKG with a P-R interval of less than 0.12 seconds and the QRS complex has an initial slur called a delta wave that broadens the complex.

There are two types of Wolff-Parkinson-White syndrome, A and B. Type B has findings similar to a left bundle branch block on an echocardiogram. There is an exaggerated diastolic dip of the interventricular septum. The appearance of type A has a brief anterior displacement of the posterior wall following electrical depolarization and may be a very subtle finding.

Ectopic rhythms such as **premature ventricular contractions (PVC's)** may alter left ventricular function due to incomplete filling. There is reduced motion of the left ventricle and interventricular septum. When PVC's occur before atrial depolarization the A wave of the mitral valve is lost in that cycle. Diastolic filling of the heart is reduced, but the left ventricular dimensions may increase since the left ventricle does not empty properly during the premature beat. Vigorous ejection and increased interventricular septal and posterior wall motion is noted during the next ventricular depolarization as a result of increased blood flow into the left ventricle.

When two PVC's occur consecutively, the D-E slope of the mitral valve is very reduced and the second complex barely has an E point. PVC's may cause reduction in the amplitude and duration of the aortic valve opening. Flattening of the interventricular septum can also occur with consecutive PVC's, or a diastolic dip just before the mitral valve opens completely and a second diastolic dip in mid systole. This is a similar appearance to that of a left bundle branch block. Measurements should never be made on a PVC or post-PVC complex.

Supraventricular tachycardia may demonstrate a large decrease in the interventricular septum and posterior wall motion. Since it is often seen with atrial fibrillation or flutter, variations in the mitral valve tracing are typically noted.

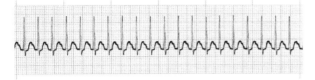

Rhythm strip of SVT

Atrial flutter causes a course anterior and posterior leaflet motion of the mitral valve, a loss of the A wave, addition of atrial flutter waves, and 2 to 1, 3 to 1 or 4 to 1 conduction. Atrial flutter is rare in adults, but common in children.

Atrial fibrillation may also cause irregular flutter of the mitral valve leaflets with loss of the A wave. Patients in Afib are at a higher risk of developing a blood clot/thrombus. The most common area for a clot/thrombus to develop is in the left atrial appendage.

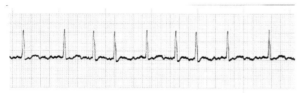

Rhythm strip of Afib

Sinus arrhythmias usually prolong the length of time the mitral valve opens, but does not affect the E to A wave.

When heart block is present or prolonged atrioventricular conduction, the echocardiographic events that depend on atrial systole will follow atrial contraction and will not be in sync with ventricular contraction. The mitral valve will close with relaxation of the atria, as well as ventricular systole. The P-R interval will be prolonged. The A wave on the mitral valve may be superimposed on the anterior leaflet during diastole and the appearance of diastolic mitral regurgitation may be noted. In a first

degree AV block, the mitral A-C interval may be prolonged and a "B bump may be seen.

On the Doppler exam a higher heart rate may cause the A velocity of the inflow tracing to follow the E velocity much closer than usual. During high heart rates the E to A velocities may become a single E/A velocity. E/A disassociation may be seen in patients with complete heart block.

Patients with atrial fibrillation have a single E wave and no A wave and are completely dependent on passive filling for cardiac output.

PARAMETERS OF LEFT VENTRICULAR FUNCTION

Contractility is the word that best describes function of the ventricle in systole. The contractility of the ventricle has many physiologic factors that can affect it. They include metabolic factors such as heart rate, coupling interval, and pharmacologic agents. Loading conditions effect left ventricular function, but may be difficult to assess with echocardiography. Preload is the initial ventricular volume or pressure and afterload is the aortic resistance or impedance, the end systolic wall stress.

Left ventricular function has typically been evaluated by echocardiography with measurements of cardiac output and ejection fraction. Left ventricular systolic function may be assessed using 2-D, M-mode and various Doppler calculations.

Terms Related to Cardiac Function

Ejection fraction is a volume measurement expressed as a percent of blood in the left ventricle in diastole ejected during systole.

Fractional shortening is a linear measurement expressed as a percent of blood in the left ventricle in diastole ejected during systole.

Cardiac output is the estimated measurement of the amount of blood ejected from the left ventricle per minute in liters.

Cardiac index is the estimated measurement of the amount of blood ejected from the left ventricle per minute in liters normalized to body surface area.

Stroke volume is the estimated measurement of the amount of blood ejected from the left ventricle per cardiac cycle.

Stroke index is the estimated measurement of the amount of blood ejected from the left ventricle per cardiac cycle normalized to body surface area. M-mode assessment of left ventricular function may be performed and is accurate in patients with normal left ventricular geometry. The short axis view at the level just past the mitral leaflet tips is typically preferred to obtain measurements. The beam should be perpendicular to the cardiac structures being evaluated. At this point measurements of the right ventricle, interventricular septum, left ventricle, and inferolateral wall (previously called posterior wall) may be made.

The American Society of Echocardiography recommends the left ventricle wall thickness and dimensions be made using the point-to-point technique.

Fractional shortening can be estimated by the following equation: Normal range is 25-44% *(Textbook of Clinical Echocardiography, 5th ed. Pg. 136).*

$$FS\% = \frac{LVIDd - LVIDs}{LVIDd} \times 100$$

LV Mass

Left ventricle mass and volumes can be calculated and used as a parameter of left ventricular function. Left ventricular mass is derived by the thickness of the walls and the left ventricle internal dimensions at end diastole. The formula to calculate left ventricular mass is:

LV mass = 0.80 x 1.05 X [(septal thickening + posterior wall thickening + left ventricle end diastole^3) - (left ventricle end diastole^3)]

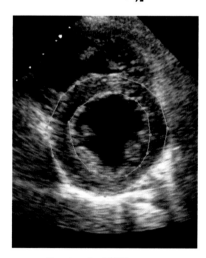

Tracing for LV Mass

225

LEFT VENTRICULAR WALL STRESS

A useful index to evaluate patients with left ventricular hypertrophy is left ventricle wall stress. This index calculates relative wall thickness. A simplified method for this estimation is:

RWT = <u>2 X posterior wall thickness</u>
Left ventricle end diastole

*RWT is relative wall thickness

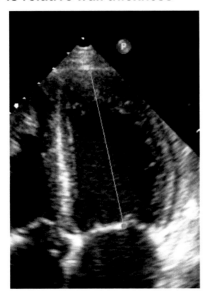

Measure LV in Apical Four Chamber

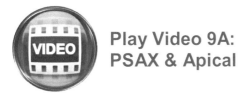

Play Video 9A:
PSAX & Apical

Ejection Fraction

Ejection fraction can be calculated using several methods, a simple equation is:

EF = (SV/EDV) X 100%

Normal EF is ≥ 52 for men and ≥ 54 women. *(Guidelines and Standards from the Journal of American Society of Echocardiography, January 2015)*

Stroke Volume

Stroke volume is calculated as:

SV = EDV-ESV

The normal ejection fraction ranges from
53 - 77%
These numbers may vary slightly among authors.

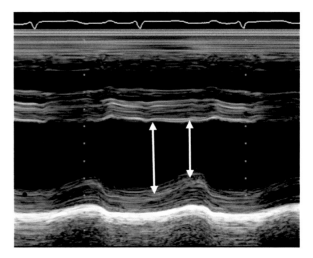

M-mode LV Systolic and Diastolic Measurements

When regional wall motion abnormalities are noted, the ejection fraction may be most accurately determined using 2-D echocardiography, heart catheterization, or radionuclide ventriculography.

Cardiac output is calculated as:

CO = SV X HR

The mean rate of circumferential fiber shortening can be measured. Since the left ventricle can be described as a series of circles, this rate helps describe the quality of the left ventricular contractions. This method is sometimes better for calculating left ventricular volume, but the measurement assumes that the left ventricle cross-sectional area is a circle.

The M-mode method uses the diameter of the ventricle which is not always shaped like a circle.

Mean rate of circumferential shortening:

mean Vcf = LVID(d) - LVID(s)
                LVID(d) X LVET

LVET is left ventricular ejection time, or the time in seconds from the point where the left ventricular posterior wall begins to move anteriorly in systole until it peaks. Measuring this in the left ventricle can be difficult. A simple, accurate measurement of left ventricular ejection time can be obtained by measuring the aortic valve from the point where it opens to the point where it closes, or on the Doppler exam from the beginning to the end of the aortic valve flow.

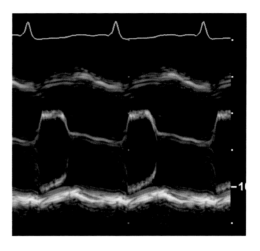

LV Ejection Time by M-mode

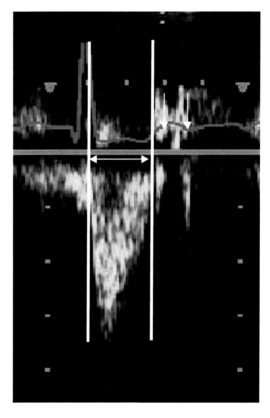

Ejection Time with Doppler

Other M-mode indications of left ventricular function are the EPSS or E point to septal separation and the degree of motion in the anterior and posterior aortic root walls.

The EPSS is measured from the E point on the mitral valve to the septum and is normally ≤ 7mm. This number may vary among authors. Normal systolic function causes the anterior mitral leaflet to open and almost fill the ventricle. When systolic dysfunction, and/or left ventricular dilation is present, this motion is reduced causing an increase in the distance of the E point to the left ventricular side of the septum.

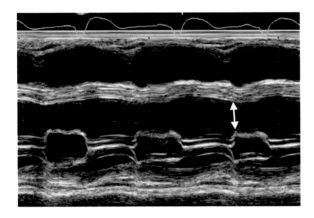

EPSS = E Point Septal Separation

The 2-D exam is usually more accurate in the estimation of left ventricular function. Multiple tomographic planes are needed, as well as good visualization of the endocardium.

Left ventricular volume can be calculated with several methods. The cubed formula is simple, but assumes that the left ventricle major axis is equal to twice the short axis dimension. This allows volume to be calculated from a single short axis view with the formula:

$$V = D^3$$

Volume can also be calculated with the single plane ellipsoid method using the length and 2-D area of the long axis view.

This can be obtained in three ways:

$$V = \frac{8A^2}{3\pi L}$$

Or

$$V = 0.85A^2/L$$

Or

$$V = (5/6\ A^2)/\ L$$

Another method to check volume is the hemicylindrical hemiellipsoid method. This assumes the left ventricle base is like a cylinder and the apex like an ellipsoid. The volume is derived by calculating the left ventricle long axis length plus cross-sectional area in short axis at the mid papillary level. The equation is:

$$V = (Am)\frac{L}{2} + \frac{2}{3}(Am)\frac{L}{2}$$

Simplification of this is the "Bullet" formula:

V = 5/6 AL

When wall motion abnormalities are present, these formulas become less accurate and volumes are usually overestimated.

Left ventricular mass can be calculated in the left ventricle short axis view at the papillary muscle level at end diastole. The endocardial and epicardial surface should be traced in its entirety. The left ventricle is measured in its longest axis in a four chamber view at end diastole.

Left ventricle myocardial mass in g/cm ^{2} is calculated as follows:

LV mass = 1.05 (total volume – chamber volume)

Simpson's rule is one of the best methods to use when regional wall motion abnormalities are present. This method uses a summation of a series of discs from the base to the apex of the left ventricle.

The MOD equation is:

$$\frac{L}{\sum (area \cdot 20)}$$

When the chamber shape is regular, less disks are needed, approximately 4-5. When it is irregular, more slices of the ventricle are necessary, at least 10 or more. This method has its problems, especially if the angle of the transducer to the left ventricle is off, or if the number of disks are not enough.

This method has been simplified or modified. The modified Simpson's rule uses three parallel slices of the left ventricle to calculate volume.

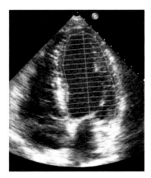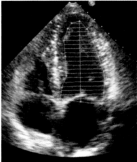

Method of Disc (MOD) or summation of discs technique

The American Society of Echocardiography recommends that the biplane apical views should be used with the modified Simpson's rule. The ventricle length is divided into twenty disks from the base to the apex. The diameter of each disk is measured in two apical views.

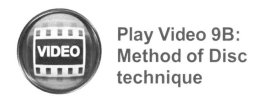

Play Video 9B: Method of Disc technique

The biggest limitation of 2-D quantification of the left ventricular function is image quality. The following techniques can help to improve the left ventricular visualization.

1. Patient positioning in a steeper left lateral decubitus position may bring cardiac structures closer to the chest wall.
2. Suppressed patient respiration or have patient exhale and hold breath.
3. Better transducer position to cardiac plane.
4. Proper gain settings to visualize the endocardium.
5. Higher frequency transducer when possible to increase resolution.
6. Adjust focus to area of interest.
7. Cineloop will help to bring in best still frame image of the heart.

Doppler calculations can be used to evaluate some left ventricular systolic functions.

Stroke volume is calculated by obtaining the cross-sectional area and velocity-time integral of flow through the region of interest. The equation is:

SV = CSA X VTI

Cross-sectional areas can be derived by obtaining a 2-D measurement of the region and using the equation:

D^2 X 0.785

229

This measurement can be done at any intracardiac site and is accurate if:

1. The cross -sectional area measurement is accurate.
2. The flow profile is spatially "flat."
3. Flow is laminar.
4. The Doppler angle is parallel to flow.
5. The diameter and velocity measurements are done at the same anatomic site.

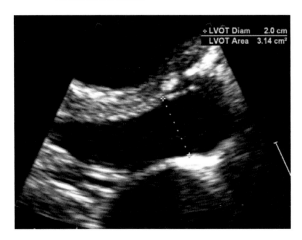

PLAX Measurement of LVOT Diameter

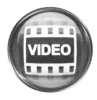 Play Video 9C: PLAX Measurement of LVOT Diameter

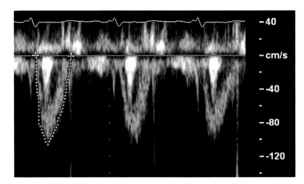

Trace LVOT flow for VTI or TVI

Cardiac output is calculated by obtaining an accurate heart rate and then using the stroke volume derived by Doppler from SV = CSA x VTI according to the following formula:

CO = HR X SV

RIGHT SIDE VOLUME OVERLOAD

There are several causes of volume overload on the right side of the heart. When a right ventricular volume overload is present, the size and shape of the right ventricle may be altered. The primary sign of right ventricular overload is typically right ventricular enlargement, however, flattening of the interventricular septum can also be an important finding.

Causes of Right Ventricular Volume Overload

- Tricuspid regurgitation
- Pulmonic regurgitation
- Shunt lesions
- Partial or total anomalous pulmonary venous connection
- Ventricular septal defect with left ventricle to right atrial shunt
- Rupture of coronary artery fistula
- Sinus of Valsalva rupture

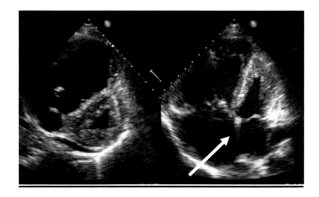

RVVO short axis and four chamber due to large atrial septal defect

 Play Video 9D: RVVO PSAX & Apical 4 due to large Atrial Septal Defect (ASD)

230

OTHER CARDIAC DIAGNOSTIC EXAMS

Cardiac Catheterization

A cardiac catheterization is a medical procedure used to diagnose and treat certain heart conditions. A thin tube called a catheter is inserted into a blood vessel in the femoral, brachial or radial artery and threaded up into the heart. A contrast agent is injected into the heart to visualize the coronary artery anatomy.

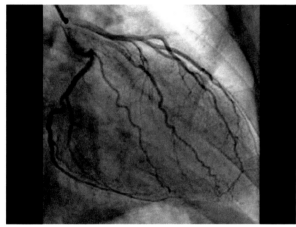

Image of coronary arteries

Heart pressures are also obtained during a cardiac catheterization. Right heart pressure waveforms can be obtained by inserting a catheter into the vein and threaded into the heart. Blood flow is antegrade as the catheter is being threaded up into the right heart to obtain right heart pressures. The catheter is inserted into the RA and a pressure is recorded, then into the RV, into the PA, and then wedged up in the pulmonary capillary level. The PCW gives an estimated LA pressure.

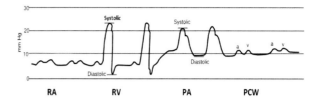

Example of Right heart pressure waveforms

A catheter can also be inserted into the artery and is threaded up into the heart to obtain left heart pressures and detect coronary artery anatomy. When inserted into the artery and threading it up the aorta, the blood flow is retrograde. The catheter is threaded up the aorta and around the aortic arch. Aortic pressure is obtained and then the catheter is threaded across the aortic valve and into the LV where a LV pressure waveform is obtained. The catheter is not threaded across the MV. The PCW pressure gives a good estimate of the LA pressure.

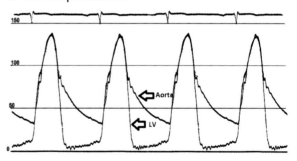

Left ventricular and Aortic pressure waveform

Abnormal pressure waveforms can be detected when obtaining this information. In mitral stenosis, LA pressure increases above normal LV diastolic pressure. A mean gradient is obtained in a cardiac catheterization in order to determine the severity of the MS.

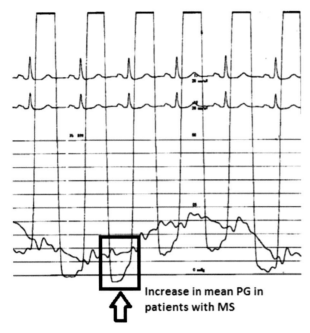

Increase in mean PG in patients with MS

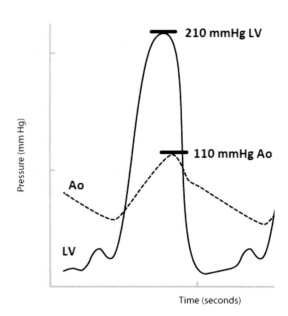

Aortic stenosis pressure waveform from cardiac cath

In patients with Aortic stenosis, the LV pressure increases and a pressure gradient is seen between the LV and Aorta. The greater the pressure gradient, the greater the degree of stenosis. Cardiac Catheterization gives a peak-to-peak gradient by simply taking the LV peak pressure and subtracting it from the peak aortic pressure. Echocardiography can also give a pressure gradient that estimates the pressure gradient across the aortic valve. Echocardiography gives an instantaneous pressure gradient versus the peak to peak gradient from cardiac catheterization.

210 – 110 = 100 mmHg PG

Nuclear Stress Test

Another diagnostic cardiac exam that is used to evaluate blood flow to the heart is known as a nuclear stress test. During the exam a small amount of radioactive tracer is injected into a vein after walking on a treadmill. A special camera, called a gamma camera, detects the radiation released by the tracer to produce computer images of the heart.

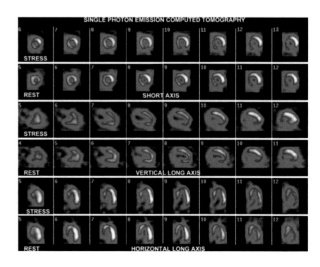

232

Magnetic Resonance Imaging

MRI is a diagnostic non-invasive exam used to diagnose and treat disease states. Using a powerful magnetic field and radio frequency pulses, detailed images of the heart are obtained.

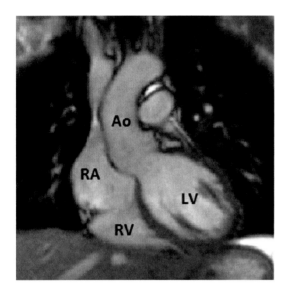

Anatomy in Cardiac MRI

Computed Tomography

Although CT obtains very similar diagnostic information as MRI, CT obtains its images using X-ray and ionized radiation.

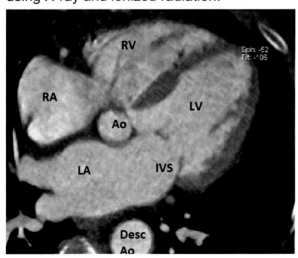

Anatomy of a CT Scan

BASIC CARDIAC PHARMACOLOGY

Although administering medication is not typically a responsibility of a cardiac sonographer, it is imperative for the sonographer to have basic knowledge of cardiac medications. Below is a list of common cardiac medications and why they are given.

Atropine- given for Sinus Bradycardia

Epinephrine- given for Cardiac Arrest, severe Sinus Bradycardia (strong inotropic and chronotropic stimulator)

Amiodarone-given for Ventricular tachycardia and Atrial fibrillation

Adenosine – given for SVT

Dobutamine – given to increase contractility (positive inotropic agent); also given in stress echo.

Dopamine -given for hypotension

Nitrates – given for Ischemic Chest pain (coronary vasodilator)

Statins -given for high cholesterol (anti hyperlipidemic)

ACE Inhibitors- given for HBP

Anticoagulants- Heparin (IV), Warfarin (PO) limits formation of thrombus

Antiplatelets- Aspirin

233

THE ROLE OF ECHO IN TRANSCATHETER AORTIC VALVE REPLACEMENT (TAVR)

Pre-op

- Baseline study with TTE provides valve anatomy, degree of calcification, quantification of severity of stenosis and LV function.

During Intervention

- TEE is performed during the procedure as a guidance when position the transcatheter valve, assess LV function after implantation and assess any complication after implantation

Post-op

- Post implantation TTE focuses on serial assessment of LV function and post- operative complication with long term use of echocardiography to assess the presence of a paravalvular leak.

THE ROLE OF ECHO IN LEFT VENTRICULAR ASSIST DEVICES

Pre-op

- TEE is used pre-operatively to assess for any cardiac contraindications for implantation of an LVAD

During procedure

- TEE assists with placement of the device including the inflow and outflow cannula, calculation of ventricular volumes and function, velocities of inflow and outflow as well as de-airing after activation.

Post-op

- Used to assess complications of LVAD's which may include intracardiac thrombosis or obstruction of inflow and outflow cannula from positioning or thrombus formation.

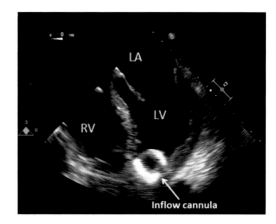

Left Ventricular Assist Device

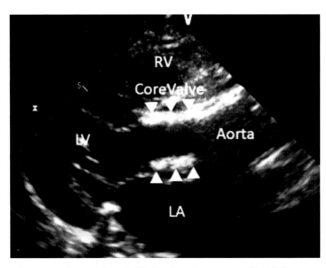

Transcatheter Aortic Valve Replacement (TAVR)

THE ROLE OF ECHO IN ASD CLOSURE DEVICES

Pre-op
- TEE provides quantification of **severity of shunt**

During procedure
- TEE is used to guide closure device for implantation

Post-op
- Assessment of complications

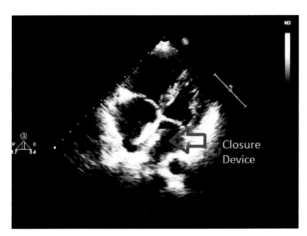

ASD Closure Device

MISCELLANEOUS QUIZ

1. The primary feature on the echocardiogram of a left bundle branch block is:
    a. upward movement of the interventricular septum at the onset of electrical depolarization
    b. downward movement of the interventricular septum at the end of electrical depolarization
    c. downward movement of the interventricular septum at the onset of electrical depolarization
    d. flattening of the interventricular septum

2. Patients with Wolff-Parkinson-White syndrome have an abnormality of the conduction rhythm that manifests itself as:
    a. premature ventricular contractions
    b. supraventricular tachycardia
    c. premature atrial contractions
    d. atrial fibrillation

3. When premature ventricular contractions occur before atrial depolarization, the tracing of the M-mode is altered by:
    a. increased A wave
    b. increased E wave
    c. loss of the A wave
    d. loss of the E wave

4. Premature ventricular contractions may cause the aortic valve opening
    a. to decrease in amplitude & duration
    b. to increase in amplitude & duration
    c. to decrease in amplitude & increase in duration
    d. to increase in amplitude & decrease in duration

5. Patients with higher than normal heart rates may cause the Doppler signal of the left ventricular inflow to:
    a. merge into a single E/A velocity
    b. have a high A velocity
    c. have a low E velocity
    d. has no effect on the E to A velocity

6. The percent of blood volume that fills the left ventricle in diastole and is ejected in systole describes:
    a. cardiac output
    b. stroke volume
    c. ejection fraction
    d. fractional shortening

7. Normal fractional shortening in adults is approximately:
    a. 60-80%
    b. 50-65%
    c. 40-65%
    d. 25-44%

8. Measuring from the opening to the closing of the aortic valve will calculate:
    a. wall stress
    b. ejection fraction
    c. left ventricular ejection time
    d. stroke volume

9. The normal EPSS should measure approximately:
    a. 2 - 7 mm
    b. 10-15 mm
    c. 15-20 mm
    d. 5-10 ms

10. The ASE recommends using the modified Simpson's rule with _____ of the left ventricle to calculate volume:
    a. 10 parallel slices + LV length
    b. 5 discs
    c. 10 discs
    d. 20 discs + LV length

11. To calculate stroke volume using Doppler in a particular region of interest, what two parameters are needed?
    a. cross-sectional area
    b. peak pressure gradient
    c. velocity time integral
    d. peak velocity
    e. a and c
    f. a and b

12. Which of the following is NOT a cause of right ventricle volume overload, RVVO?
    a. Shunts like ASD's & VSD's
    b. Pulmonic regurgitation
    c. Tricuspid Regurgitation
    d. Pericardial effusions

13. The following M-mode is a measurement of:
    a. EF slope
    b. DE excursion
    c. MV ejection time
    d. EPSS

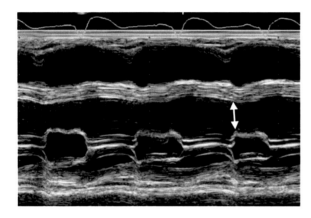

14. The following is a diagnostic image of:
    a. Nuclear stress test
    b. Magnetic Resonance Imaging
    c. Cardiac Catheterization
    d. Computed Tomography

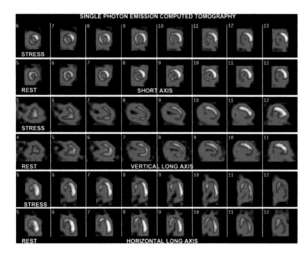

15. Name the anatomy in the following image marked by an "X":
    a. LV
    b. Aorta
    c. Pulmonary artery
    d. IVC

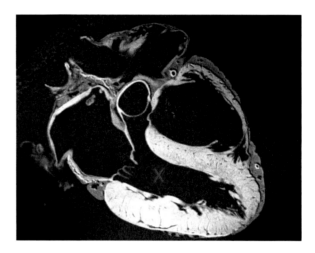

16. What medication is used in stress echo if a patient cannot walk on a treadmill?
    a. Dopamine
    b. Atropine
    c. Dobutamine
    d. Epinephrine

17. ACE inhibitors are used to treat:
    a. Arrhythmias
    b. Congestive Heart Failure
    c. High Blood Pressure
    d. Atrial Fibrillation

18. Patient in Atrial fibrillation are commonly on this medication to help reduce the formation of a blood clot:
    a. ACE Inhibitor
    b. Statin
    c. Anticoagulant
    d. Anti-arrhythmic

19. Statins are used for:
    a. high blood pressure
    b. high cholesterol
    c. high heart rate
    d. high cardiac output

20. Diagnose the cardiac cath pressure waveform:
    a. Aortic stenosis
    b. Mitral stenosis
    c. Cardiac tamponade
    d. Pulsus paradoxus

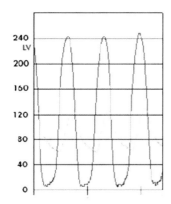

21. Diagnose the cardiac cath pressure waveform:
    a. Aortic stenosis
    b. Mitral stenosis
    c. Cardiac tamponade
    d. Pulsus paradoxus

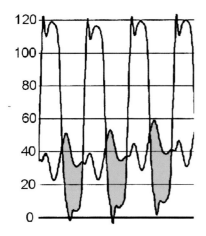

22. What pressure waveform is the best estimate of the LA pressure?
    a. Right ventricle
    b. Right atrial
    c. Pulmonary artery
    d. Pulmonary capillary wedge

23. What diagnostic exam is seen in the image below?
    a. Nuclear stress test
    b. Magnetic resonance imaging
    c. Cardiac catheterization
    d. Computed tomography

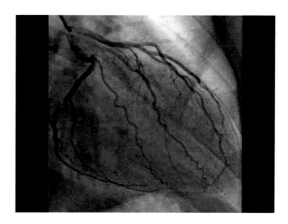

24. What is being measured in the Doppler image below:
    a. Peak LVOT velocity
    b. LV ejection time
    c. Rapid filling time
    d. None of the above

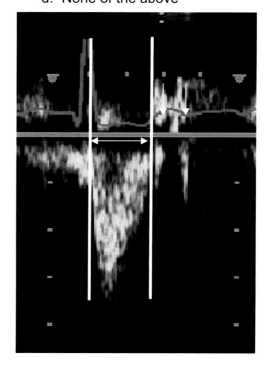

25. Diagnose the following arrhythmia:

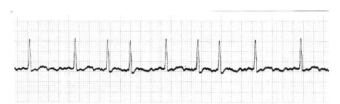

    a. Atrial fibrillation
    b. Ventricular tachycardia
    c. Left bundle branch block
    d. Sinus bradycardia

26. Which type of pressure gradient across the aortic valve is obtained from echocardiography:
    a. peak-to-peak
    b. alternating
    c. continuous
    d. instantaneous

27. What is the treatment of choice for the following arrhythmia:

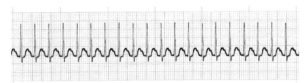

    a. adenosine
    b. epinephrine
    c. statin
    d. atropine

28. What is the treatment of choice for severe bradycardia or asystole?
    a. adenosine
    b. lasix
    c. atropine
    d. beta blocker

Section 10:

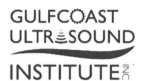

Congenital Heart Disease In the Adult

Section 10: CONGENITAL HT DISEASE IN THE ADULT

Objectives

Upon completion of this module you should be able to:

- Identify various types of congenital heart diseases found in adults

- Recognize the types of aortic stenosis

- State the etiologies of congenital heart disease

- Recognize the types of atrial and septal defects and their associated findings

- Apply the echocardiographic methods to evaluate cardiac shunts, valvular stenosis, and related regurgitant lesions

- Relate knowledge of normal cardiac hemodynamics to the abnormal effects of the various congenital heart diseases

BASIC EMBRYOLOGY

PRIMITIVE HEART TUBE

Early in embryonic cardiovascular development, a pair of heart tubes is formed from the primitive vascular system of the fetus. A section of the main vascular channel specializes and develops contractile properties within its vessel walls. These heart tubes lie parallel to each other and in close proximity at the cephalic end of the fetus. Eventually, the pair of heart tubes fuses into a single endocrinal tube that retains its contractile properties. The wall of the primitive heart tube consists of an external myocardial mantle 1 to 2 cell layers thick. In addition, the wall also consists of a single layer of endothelial cells and is separated from the myocardial mantle by a basically structure less, cellular, third layer called cardiac jelly. The primordial heart is developed from the heart tube. The heart tube can be separated into chambers. The sinus venous is located caudally at the inflow portion, followed by the primitive atria, the ventricles, and the bulbous cords, which is the most cranially located.

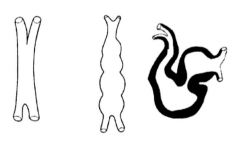

Primitive heart tube

Sinus venosus

In the embryo, the **sinus venosus** is a separate chamber from the fetal common atria. It is made up of the following structures:

- central, unpaired portion
- transverse portion,
- right sinus horn
- left sinus horn

Each of these structures in the embryonic heart develops into or becomes incorporated into structures which make up the adult heart. The left horn of the sinus venosus forms the coronary sinus, while the right horn becomes absorbed into the right atrium as the sinus venarum, into which the great veins open. In addition, small folds appear on the right side of the sinus venosus which become the left and right sinus valves. The left sinus valve then fuses with the atrial septum and the right sinus valve forms the **Eustachian and thebesian valves**.

Cardiac loop

At approximately day 23 in embryonic development, the growing heart tube is referred to as the **bulboventricular tube,** and bends to the right and anteriorly to form a sigmoid shape. This process is called **cardiac looping** and is believed to be a fundamental and intrinsic property of the myocardium, rather than a space saving adaptation in the rapidly growing fetus. At the same time and considered a part of cardiac looping, the aortic arches are developed in the cephalic portion of the bulboventricular tube. At the caudal half of the heart tube, tissue expansion forms the early version of the adult ventricle. The primitive atria lie extra pericardial and caudal to the ventricles. Looping adds a certain amount of torsion to the developing heart which is responsible in part for the spiral disposition of the interventricular septum.

Aortic arches

In the fetus, simultaneous with cardiac looping is a process which results in the formation of six arches which make up the aortic arch system.

These arches develop from the aortic sac portion of the primitive heart tube and come and go with the ever- changing structures of the fetal heart. These six arches are functional although only arches number three, four, and six persist in the adult heart and become the following:

- Number three becomes the carotid arteries
- Number four forms the aortic arch
- Number six forms the pulmonary arteries and ductus arteriosus

Septation

Cardiac septation is the process dividing the rapidly growing and expanding portions of the heart tube into the four distinct chambers of the adult heart. Septation takes place more or less simultaneously with the development of the primitive ventricles, conus cordis, and truncus arteriosus.

Septation is the result of three mechanisms

1. **Passive septation** is the fusing together of the growing and expanding wall segments of the primitive heart chambers.

2. **Active septation** is the growth of a layer of cardiac mesenchyme called endocardial cushion tissue. This tissue is derived from the earlier cardiac jelly and grows new cells which fuse together to form parts of the septa in the heart.

3. The third process of septation is a **combination** of the first two methods. This method starts out as passive septation only to have growth completed by endocardial tissue along borders which grow and fuse together.

Partitioning of the embryonic heart is completed by the formation of seven septa, three of which are passively formed, three

of which are actively formed, and one that is formed by a combination of both methods.

Valve formation

Valve formation in the embryonic heart is accomplished primarily by infolding and growth of the muscular ventricular wall which is facilitated by the process of **diverticulation**. The remaining growth is completed by the expansion and fusion of endocardial tissue. Early in the development of the atrioventricular valves, they are thick and fleshy only to transform into the thin, fibrous cusps seen in the adult.

COMPARISON OF FETAL AND POSTNATAL CIRCULATION

Upon completion of the embryonic development of the fetal heart, there are still a few differences that stand out from the postnatal state. Fetal cardiovascular needs are met by certain modifications that differentiate it from post natal circulation. In the fetus, highly oxygenated blood returns from the placenta in the umbilical vein. Half of this blood passes through the fetal liver and the other half through the inferior vena cava via the **ductus venosus**. After a short course through the inferior vena cava, the saturated blood enters the right atrium. The saturated blood is mixed with desaturated blood returning from the superior vena cava.

The design of the right atrium directs the majority of saturated blood through the **foramen ovale** into the fetal left atrium. A small percentage of the mixed, but still highly-saturated blood, crosses the tricuspid valve, passes into the right ventricle, and is ejected out of the pulmonary artery. Some of the blood goes to the lungs, but the majority is shunted to the descending aorta through the **ductus arteriosus**.

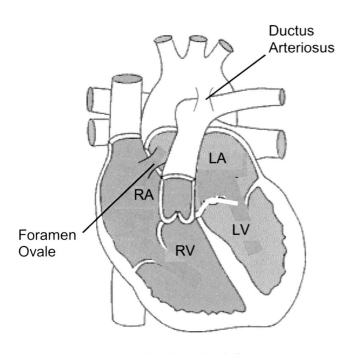

Cardiac fetal circulation

Shortly after birth the three shunts present in the fetal circulation cease to function. The ductus venosus constricts so all blood entering the liver must pass through the hepatic sinusoids. Occlusion of the placental circulation causes an immediate fall in blood pressure in the inferior vena cava and right atrium. Aeration of the lungs with the first breath causes a dramatic fall in pulmonary vascular resistance and an increase in pulmonary blood flow. The second shunt closes when increased pulmonary blood flow causes left atrial pressure to rise, closing the flap of the foramen ovale. The third shunt is the ductus arteriosus which constricts at birth with the presence of bradykinins. Bradykinins is a substance released in the lungs with their initial inflation.

It is important to remember that the change from fetal to adult circulation is a gradual occurrence that often occurs over weeks. During the transitional stage there is often some flow through the three fetal circulatory structures.

During the complex stage of embryologic development of the heart, congenital lesions may develop which may or may not constitute a serious threat to life. Approximately 8 per 1000 live births result in some kind of congenital cardiac abnormality. Of these births, about 1/3 or 2.6 per 1000 births manifest critical heart disease.

The most common explanation as to why congenital defects occur is that they are due to a combination of genetics and environmental interactions. Risk to the fetus is increased with a genetic predisposition, as well as exposure to an environmental teratogen during a critical or vulnerable period of development. Children of parents with certain types of congenital defects are at a higher risk, with an approximately 8.8% chance of developing significant cardiac lesions.

ABNORMALITIES OF SEPTATION

Congenital cardiac defects in the newborn can be classified into four categories:

1. Abnormalities of septation
2. Abnormal vasculature
3. Valvular abnormalities
4. Persistence of fetal circulation

A ventricular septal defect is the most common abnormality, followed by pulmonary stenosis, patent ductus arteriosus, atrial septal defect (secundum type), and aortic stenosis

Abnormalities of Septation (Atrial)

There are three types of atrial septal defects which are classified as to their location, they are: **venosus**, **secundum**, and **primum** defects. The atrial septum is divided into three regions based on embryologic derivation of the area.

A **sinus venosus atrial septal defect** is located at the most superior portion of the atrial septum. It is bordered by the posterior wall of atria, the right atrial appendage, and the limbus of the fossa ovale. It lies in close proximity to the right sided pulmonary veins and superior vena cava. This defect is sometimes associated with anomalous pulmonary venous return.

A **secundum or fossa ovalis defect** is the most common atrial septal defect. It is located inferior and anterior to the sinus venosus region. The secundum region is the thinnest portion of the atrial septum and is composed of the flap which covers the foramen ovale.

Primum or atrioventricular defect is bordered by the atrioventricular valves, posterior atrial wall, and the fossa ovalis. Primum defects are usually part of a complex anomaly involving AV canal defects.

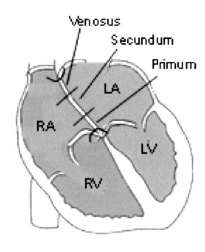

Location of atrial septal defects

Abnormalities of Septation (Ventricular)

The other types of septal defects are termed ventricular septal defects. The ventricular septum is divided into two major parts, the membranous and muscular portions. The **membranous septum** is relatively small, thin, and centrally located in the heart. It is bounded superiorly by the aortic valve and at the junction of the right and noncoronary cusps, and inferiorly by the muscular septum.

The **muscular septum** fans out from the membranous septum and lies inferior. There are three components to the muscular septum: **the inlet portion, the orbicular septum, and the outlet septum**. Cardiac defects can occur at any one of these points and are defined by their location.

Abnormal Vasculature and Resulting Lesions

In addition to defects in cardiac septation, the embryologic heart may develop abnormal vasculature and communication between cardiac structures. Some of the more well-known include the following:

- Patent Ductus Arteriosus
- Anomalous Pulmonary Venous Return
- Coarctation of the Aorta
- Transposition of the Great Arteries
- Truncus Arteriosus

Anomalous pulmonary venous return involves the effective attachment of one or more of the pulmonary veins to some other structure other than the left atrium.

Coarctation of the aorta is an abnormal narrowing of this vessel usually just beyond the left subclavian artery.

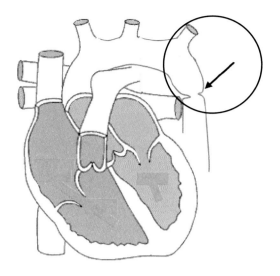

Coarctation of the Aorta

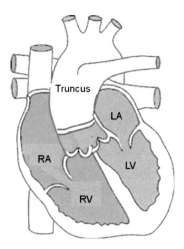

Truncus Arteriosus

Transposition of the great arteries is an abnormal connection of the aorta and pulmonary artery to their respective ventricles.

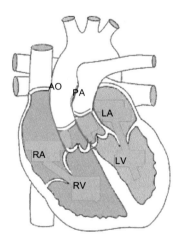

Transposition of the Great Arteries

Truncus Arteriosus involves a defect where the aorta and pulmonary artery fail to separate from their common origin and result in a single vessel being fed from both ventricles.

Persistence of Normal Fetal Communication

There are two main types of defects caused by persistent fetal circulation in the natal state: patent ductus arteriosus, and patent foramen ovale.

Patent Ductus Arteriosus is the persistence of the communication between the aorta and the main pulmonary artery.

Patent Foramen Ovale is the continued patency of the fossa ovales resulting in communication of blood flow between the right and left atrium.

Valvular Anomalies

Congenital heart defects can be primarily valvular in origin, as well as in combination with the cardiac defects mentioned previously. Valvular abnormalities in the newborn can take one of four forms. The diseased valve may be **atretic** meaning missing altogether, it may be **hypoplastic** or underdeveloped, it may be **intrinsically stenotic**, or it may have some malformation of its leaflets which cause it to be **regurgitant, stenotic**, or **both.**

A **bicuspid aortic valve** is one of the most common congenital heart defects. The normal aortic valve has three cusps. In this congenital defect, the aortic valve has two cusps. Bicuspid aortic valves tend to become stenotic, but can be regurgitant. Bicuspid valves are at a much greater risk of developing endocarditis. Other common forms of congenital valvular heart disease include: **tricuspid atresia**, **truncus arteriosus**, a situation with a common semilunar valve, and **pulmonary atresia**.

Less common, but of note is **Ebstein's anomaly** and cleft mitral valve. **Ebstein's anomaly** is the apical displacement of the septal and posterior leaflets of the tricuspid valve. It results in the atrialization of the proximal portion of the right ventricle. It is a cyanotic heart lesion and is associated with right ventricular conduction delays, right ventricular bundle branch block, and Wolf-Parkinson-White syndrome.

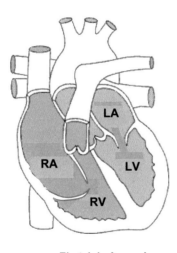

Ebstein's Anomaly

Cleft mitral valve is a formation of the mitral valve where a split develops in the anterior leaflet and is associated with other defects of the **atrioventricular canal**. It is usually associated with a large degree of mitral insufficiency.

A **parachute mitral valve** is one in which both leaflets of the mitral valve insert into one papillary muscle. This commonly results in mitral stenosis, with associated left sided systemic stenosis.

CONGENITAL HEART DISEASE IN THE ADULT

Categories

In adult echocardiography two basic areas of congenital heart disease are found. They are patients who present with undiagnosed, untreated congenital problems and patients who have had, or have known defects, either treated or not and survived into adulthood.

Both areas are challenging for the echocardiographer. In the patient who has had previous intervention, post-operative anatomy, progressing anomalies, and residual effects need to be determined. In the undiagnosed patient, the correct abnormality and recognition of it is important for proper treatment.

Bicuspid aortic valve is the most common congenital heart defect and occurs in 1-2% of the population. Patients are not usually affected until age 50-60. The bicuspid valve has two cusps instead of the normal three. It is often associated with coarctation of the aorta, a narrowing of the aorta.

Coarctation is usually located distal to the origin of the left subclavian artery. The cusps in a bicuspid valve are usually unequal in size, one cusp may have a raphe (typically the larger cusp). A raphe is a crease or seam and may appear as a third cusp best visualized during systole in the parasternal short axis view. The bicuspid valve may become stenotic in adults and may not be discovered until the stenosis becomes significant. Patients with a bicuspid valve have a higher risk for endocarditis and aortic regurgitation.

There are two types of bicuspid valves. With type I the cusps are located anteriorly and posteriorly. The coronary arteries arise anterior to the anterior cusp and the commissures are right and left. In type II, the cusps attach right and left with anterior and posterior commissures. The coronary arteries arise from behind each cusp.

On the 2-D exam the bicuspid valve may have systolic bowing of the leaflets into the aorta on the parasternal long axis view. Cusps may appear thick, if not calcific, and eccentric closure may be noted. On the parasternal short axis view during systole, instead of the normal triangular appearance of the aortic valve excursion, the valve opening appears oval or round.

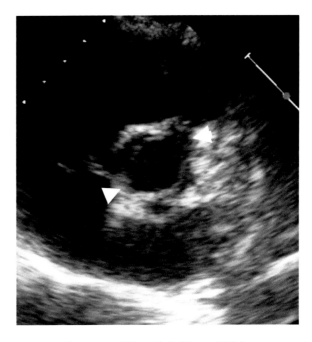

Parasternal Short Axis Bicuspid Valve

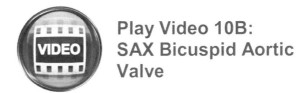

Play Video 10B: SAX Bicuspid Aortic Valve

The M-mode exam may show the decreased valve excursion if stenosis is present. Eccentric closure of the valve may be noted. If closure of the valve is 1/3 or greater from the midline of the aortic root or the eccentricity index is 1.3 or greater, abnormal cusp location is suggested. Approximately 25% of patients with bicuspid valves have a normal eccentricity index. False positive findings may result if the transducer is improperly positioned.

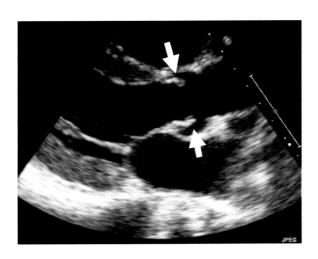

Parasternal Long Axis Bicuspid Valve

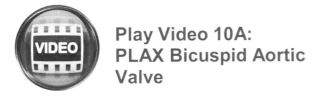

Play Video 10A: PLAX Bicuspid Aortic Valve

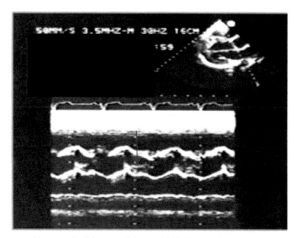

Eccentric Closure Bicuspid Valve on M-mode

The Doppler exam of a bicuspid valve may reveal aortic stenosis and regurgitation. The most common associated abnormality is coarctation of the aorta, however, in a small percent of cases ventricular septal defects have occurred.

Supravalvular aortic stenosis or stenosis above the valve is usually a result of a congenital fibrous band or constriction, usually located just above the valve level. This condition may occur sporadically, but may be familial. It is associated with William's syndrome. **William's syndrome** is characterized by mental retardation, supravalvular stenosis, a high, prominent forehead, epicanthal folds, overhanging upper lip, and an undeveloped nose bridge and mandible.

The clinical findings in patients with a supravalvular stenosis are a prominent systolic thrill in the carotid arteries and suprasternal notch, as well as a systolic ejection murmur. There may be a difference in systolic blood pressures between the arms.

On the 2-D exam the parasternal long axis view may show the defect. There may be left ventricular hypertrophy with normal left ventricular function. The aortic valve is usually normal. Pulse wave Doppler interrogation should be directed superior to the defect to accurately localize the stenosis while continuous wave Doppler should quantify the severity.

Subvalvular aortic stenosis may result from several different conditions. There are three basic types of subvalvular stenosis. Type I occurs when a fibrous type collar encircles the left ventricular outflow tract a short distance below the valve usually 1 to 1.5 cm. from the aortic valve level. The anterior mitral leaflet may be involved in the attachment of the membrane. Type II is a muscular deformity of the interventricular septum in the subaortic region. Type III is the least common type and is a fibromuscular tunnel or tunnel subaortic stenosis.

The subvalvular portion of the left ventricular outflow tract is usually fibrotic with frequent involvement of the anterior mitral leaflet. Left ventricular outflow tract narrowing is extensive. The aortic annulus and ascending aorta may be hypoplastic.

2-D imaging may be helpful in the differentiation of the types of subvalvular stenosis, especially using the parasternal long axis and apical five chamber views. Left ventricular hypertrophy may be an associated finding.

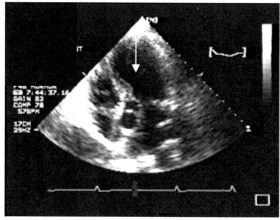

Subvalvular Stenosis Apical Five Chamber

The use of color flow imaging helps with the location of flow disturbances typically located on the left ventricular side of the valve. Aortic regurgitation may coexist due to the chronic exposure to the high velocity flow.

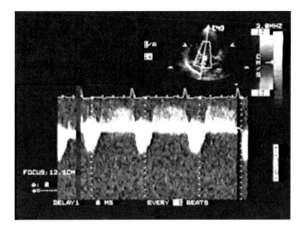

Doppler subvalvular stenosis and associated aortic regurgitation

Pulmonic stenosis is somewhat rare and often associated with Tetralogy of Fallot, but may be an isolated finding. Pulmonic stenosis can occur at three levels: valvular, infundibular, or in the pulmonary arterial system

Stenosis at the valve level may show thickened cusps with systolic bowing. The pulmonary trunk may be dilated as compared to the valve itself. Pulmonary artery pressures are usually lower than usual, however, the right ventricular pressure will be elevated. Doppler distal to the obstruction is high velocity, and pulmonic regurgitation may be present.

Pulmonic stenosis at the **infundibular level** or outflow tract is usually caused by a fibrous band or ring, or hypertrophy of the subvalvular muscle. Isolated infundibular stenosis is rare and is often secondary to Tetralogy of Fallot, valvular pulmonic stenosis, or right ventricular muscle bundle.

Supravalvular pulmonic stenosis may occur as a result of coarctation of the pulmonary

arterial system. It is most commonly associated with downstream obstruction and infants having had the fetal infection of rubella. Rubella infected patients may also have a patent ductus arteriosus. Occasionally, coarctation of the pulmonary artery is associated with supravalvular aortic stenosis or coarctation of the aorta.

Recordings of the peak pressure gradient should be made in patients with pulmonic stenosis and pulmonic valve area determinations if possible. Remember to check for pulmonic regurgitation. Right ventricular hypertrophy may be present since pulmonic stenosis has a high association with Tetralogy of Fallot. Check for a ventricular septal defect and overriding aorta.

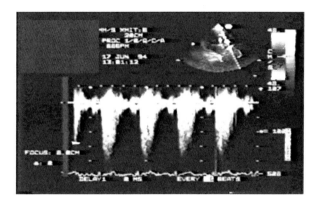

Doppler of Pulmonic Stenosis

Cleft mitral valve is an abnormality of the anterior mitral leaflet that is a common finding in atrioventricular canal or endocardial cushion defect.

The parasternal long and short axis view may be most helpful to determine cleft mitral valve. Mitral regurgitation is common and color flow imaging and pulsed Doppler techniques are helpful for identification.

Atrial septal defects are abnormal communications or holes in the interatrial septum. They are the second most common form of congenital defects in adults. They are classified according to position in the interatrial septum and to embryologic origin. Approximately 50% of patients with these defects are asymptomatic. Symptoms are often relative to the amount of the left to right shunting of blood flow and pulmonary resistance.

When there is an abnormal communication in the septum, blood flow will shunt from left to right or from high pressure to low pressure. When the right side pressure becomes higher the shunt will change to a right to left shunt. If patients are symptomatic, dyspnea, palpitations, and arrhythmia's may occur. Pulmonary hypertension may be present, as well as a systolic ejection murmur, and possible fixed splitting of the 2nd heart sound. There are five types of atrial septal defects: ostium secundum, sinus venosus, and ostium primum, unroofed coronary sinus, and common atrium.

Atrial secundum defects are those located in the region of the fossa ovalis. These occur as a result of failure of development of the septum secundum. They are the most common and are responsible for approximately 70% of all atrial septal defects.

Sinus venosus defects are located high in the atrial septum near the entrance of the superior vena cava. These account for approximately 6-8% of atrial septal defects and may be associated with abnormal drainage of the right pulmonary vein.

Ostium primum defects are located anterior to the os of the coronary sinus. The lower margins of the defect are continuous with the atrioventricular valves. These make up about 20% of all atrial septal defects and are the partial form of common atrioventricular canal.

Other very rare areas for atrial septal defects to occur are the posterior and inferior entrance of the inferior vena cava or the region of the coronary sinus or a complete absence of the atrial septum.

The size of the atrial septal defect can range from a few millimeters to 3cm or greater. Usually defects of 1cm or greater are of clinical significance.

A **patent foramen ovale** is not considered a true atrial septal defect since it is guarded on the left atrial side by a flap of tissue from the septum primum. This flap prevents shunting unless left atrial pressure or size increases and causes the flap to become incompetent.

2-D imaging for atrial septal defects can be obtained from several views. The subcostal approach is the best way to visualize the atrial septum as it courses perpendicular to the ultrasound beam from this approach.

The parasternal short axis may help to show the defect, but typically the subcostal views provide the best imaging and Doppler planes. The apical views should be avoided as artifacts and "drop out" are common. When shunting is from the left to right, high velocity, turbulent flow may be seen through the defect and into the right atrium. If the shunt is significant, right atrial and ventricular enlargement occurs and paradoxical septal motion is possible due to the right ventricular volume overload. The abnormal septal motion and right ventricular volume overload may sometimes be the first indication that a patient has an atrial septal defect.

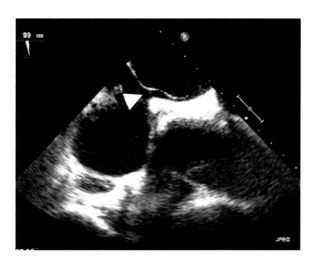

Patent Foramen Ovale with Incompetent Flap due to increased left atrial pressure in TEE image

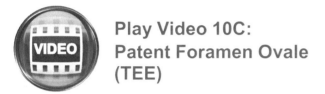

Play Video 10C:
Patent Foramen Ovale
(TEE)

Color flow imaging is helpful in determining the location, timing, and direction of flow. Flow from the superior vena cava often streams along the interatrial septum and may cause confusion or false findings. The pulmonary to systemic shunt ratio or **QP/QS** can be quantified by Doppler. Measurements of stroke volume at the aortic and pulmonary valves is needed.

In an atrial septal defect, the transpulmonic volume or QP is obtained from the cross-sectional area of the pulmonary artery and the VTI of the outflow. The systemic volume flow or Qs is obtained from the cross-sectional area of the left ventricular outflow tract and a VTI of the outflow tract flow. QP:Qs = CSA(pa) x VTI(pa) /CSA (lvot) x VTI(lvot). Patients with a QP/Qs of greater than 2:1 are usually symptomatic.

The pulmonary artery flow should be evaluated in these patients for increased velocity flow and for pulmonary hypertension. **The right ventricular systolic pressure** can be measured by using the equation RVSP= $4V^2$ +RAP (tricuspid velocity jet is V^2).

Agitated saline echo can be performed to detect left to right shunting. Agitated saline echo is performed by injecting agitated saline into the peripheral venous flow. Microbubbles should be seen across the interatrial septum even in a left to right shunt since there is a short time when right atrial pressure exceeds left atrial pressure. This is done more commonly to detect right to left shunts, especially in patients with a patent foramen ovale having systemic embolic events or to determine the potential for them.

Patients' having echocardiograms who have had repairs of their defects should be carefully evaluated. Mild right atrial and ventricular dilatation may be present, but anything more is suspicious for a residual defect or a leak in or around the patch.

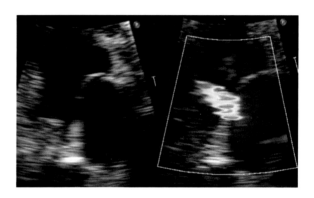

CFI of Atrial Septal Defect

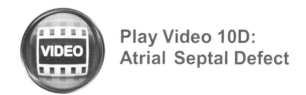

Play Video 10D:
Atrial Septal Defect

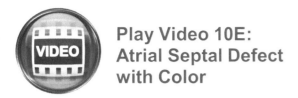

Play Video 10E:
Atrial Septal Defect
with Color

Ventricular septal defects are abnormal connections or holes in the interventricular septum. It can be an isolated defect or can also occur with other cardiac defects.

Patients with ventricular septal defects will have varying symptoms based on the size of the defect, the amount of left to right shunting, and the pulmonary vascular resistance. If symptomatic, the patients may have a systolic murmur, enlarged heart, congestive heart failure, and dyspnea. Ventricular septal defects, atrial septal defects, and patent ductus arteriosus are more prone to endocarditis.

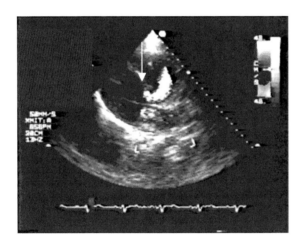

CFI Ventricular Septal Defect associated with Tetralogy of Fallot

Ventricular septal defects can be divided into two types of defects: supracristal and infracristal defects.

Supracristal defects lie just below the pulmonic valve and **infracristal defects** lie inferior and posterior to the crista supraventricularis. These defects are further divided into membranous, muscular, inlet, and outlet ventricular septal defects.

Membranous ventricular septal defects are the most common and are located in the membranous interventricular septum. This is inferomedial to the aortic valve and lateral to the tricuspid septal leaflet. These may close spontaneously during childhood. A ventricular septal aneurysm may result at the site.

Muscular interventricular defects are located at any location in the muscular interventricular septum and can be small and difficult to detect. Generally, these defects are located anterior, mid, posterior, or apically.

Inlet defects are in the sinus portion of the interventricular septum, slightly inferior to the aortic valve plane, and next to the annulus of the mitral and tricuspid valves. These are often associated with other abnormalities such as primum atrial septal defects, atrioventricular valve abnormalities, or a complete atrioventricular canal defect.

Supracristal ventricular septal defects are rarely diagnosed in adults. These are located in the right ventricular outflow past the interventricular septum. These defects are sometimes referred to as outlet, or subpulmonary defects.

2-D findings of a ventricular septal defect may be difficult when the defect is less than 3mm. Even when shunts are left to right, the left side of the heart will most likely be enlarged. This is due to the fact that there is actually a bigger return of flow to the left, causing left sided enlargement. Aortic valve prolapse may be present. As discussed previously, an aneurysm may be seen in the interventricular septum, especially at the site of a previously repaired defect. If shunts are large, Eisenmenger's physiology may occur resulting in right to left shunts with right ventricular dilatation and hypertrophy. **Eisenmenger's syndrome or physiology** results when there is a left to right shunt that develops severe pulmonary vascular disease that causes pulmonary resistance to become higher than systemic resistance. This causes blood flow shunting to be predominately right to left.

Eisenmenger's complex refers to a congenital cyanotic heart defect consisting of a ventricular septal defect, dextroposition of the aorta, pulmonary hypertension, pulmonary artery enlargement, and right ventricular hypertrophy.

Pulsed wave Doppler should be directed towards the right ventricular side of the interventricular septum if a left to right shunt is suspected. If a right to left shunts is present, Doppler detection is made from the left ventricular side of the interventricular septum. Color flow imaging is very helpful for the detection of these defects. The parasternal long axis, possibly the short axis, apical, and subcostal views provide excellent sites for interrogation.

The peak pressure gradient of the shunt can be obtained from the peak velocity of the shunt flow and applying it to the modified Bernoulli equation. The Qp/Qs ratio is usually normal in adults with ventricular septal defects since the defects are typically small, but the measurement should still be obtained. The same procedure should be followed to obtain systemic and pulmonic output as with the atrial septal defect.

On the Doppler exam the right ventricle pressure may be estimated by using the formula:

RVP = Systolic blood pressure - ventricular septal defect shunt gradient.

The shunt gradient is calculated by applying the modified Bernoulli equation. The **ductus arteriosus** is a vascular channel that is necessary in fetal circulation and usually closes 2-3 weeks after birth. When it does not close, it is referred to as a **patent ductus arteriosus** and a left to right shunt occurs from the aorta to the main pulmonary artery near the take-off of the left pulmonary artery. If the left ventricle compensates, usually due to the fact that aortic pressure is not fully transmitted to the pulmonary artery pressure, then the patient may remain stable for years. Occlusive

pulmonary vascular disease may occur and a right to left shunt can result.

Patent ductus arteriosus is hard to detect in adults due to the location. The parasternal short axis view and right inflow view may be helpful. The patient may have an enlarged left ventricle and left atrium due to the chronic overload if a left to right shunt is present.

The Doppler exam may work best for the detection of this abnormality through the location of the shunt flow. Flow in the pulmonary artery should be sampled to detect the disturbed flow. Pulmonic regurgitation is also possible. Holodiastolic flow reversal may be noted in the descending aorta as a result of antegrade flow into the ductus during diastole and must be differentiated from diastolic flow reversal due to severe aortic regurgitation.

Endocardial cushion defects (or atrioventricular canal defects) are located at an area where the atrial and ventricular septa meet the mitral and tricuspid valves. These types of defects have a high incidence in Down's syndrome. When the defect is complete the following abnormalities are present: a primum atrial septal defect, a ventricular septal defect, and clefts of both the mitral and tricuspid valves. If the defect is incomplete there is an ostium or underdeveloped primum atrial septal defect and cleft mitral valve. The interventricular septum is usually normal, as well as the tricuspid valve, although, some tricuspids valves may be cleft. Since the attachments to the interventricular septum are abnormal, the anterior mitral leaflet is displaced into the left ventricular outflow tract resulting in an opening superiorly. A helpful method of understanding the classifications is as follows:

1. Complete - large VSD
2. Transitional - restrictive VSD
3. Incomplete - no VSD

The parasternal view of this region shows the narrowed left ventricular outflow tract. In a complete defect the ventricular septal defect is located just below the

257

atrioventricular ring and is continuous with the atrial septal defect.

2-D and M-mode findings may show paradoxical septal motion, an abnormal mitral valve closure with a thick anterior leaflet, and possibly a dilated right ventricle, unless a ventricular septal defect is present.

If large enough, the atrial and ventricular septal defects should be seen, and the septal tricuspid leaflet and the anterior mitral leaflet may be formed as one leaflet.

The Doppler interrogation should be performed for the various defects and gradients and shunt ratio's calculated.

Ebstein's anomaly is a downward displacement of the septal and occasionally the posterior leaflets of the tricuspid valve. This results in a decreased right ventricle size and an increased right atrial size. The portion of the right ventricle that is below the abnormal valve becomes "atrialized" and acts as a receiving chamber. The anterior leaflet is usually the largest and least affected, while involvement of the septal or posterior leaflet is more commonly seen. The posterior leaflet may be absent or rudimentary. Secondary findings may include: secundum atrial septal defects or the interatrial septum may have an incomplete or fenestrated foramen ovale.

Three factors affect the right heart causing it to be abnormal in this disease: the malformation of the tricuspid valve, the atrialized right ventricle, and the reduction in the capacity of the pumping portion of the right ventricle. Symptoms may include: fatigue, dyspnea, right sided congestive heart failure, arrhythmias, atrial fibrillation, and Wolff-Parkinson-White syndrome.

The apical view usually shows the abnormal tricuspid valve and atrialized right ventricle. Tricuspid regurgitation will be present with the amounts depending on the severity of the disease and septal motion may be flattened or paradoxical.

Tetralogy of Fallot is a congenital disease with four primary characteristics: a membranous ventricular septal defect, the aorta is large and overrides the ventricular septal defect, and there is a right ventricular outflow tract obstruction that can be valvular, sub-valvular, or supravalvular. Right ventricular hypertrophy may be present as a secondary finding to the large VSD and systemic RV pressures. Subclinical Tetralogy of Fallot is rarely seen in adults due to the high mortality rate. Symptoms may include dyspnea, syncope, and cyanosis in the untreated patient.

The 2-D exam in the parasternal long axis view shows the enlarged, overriding aorta. If the ventricular septal defect has been patched, then that area may appear increased in echogenicity.
The short axis right ventricular outflow tract view should be used to determine pulmonic stenosis with the Doppler. Check for a possible patent ductus arteriosus. Color flow imaging and Doppler are helpful for detecting abnormal jets due to stenosis or shunts from leaking patches or residual septal defects.

Coarctation of the aorta is a congenital narrowing of the aorta usually occurring in the proximal descending aorta just above the ductus arteriosus. The narrowing can be long or only a short segment can be affected. The suprasternal view may be most helpful in detecting coarctation.

Doppler of an unoperated coarctation may be difficult since jets are often eccentric. Doppler performed on patients with previous surgical repair that have restenosed, may result in more symmetrical jets and easier detection. Coarctation may be seen in conjunction with other defects such as a bicuspid aortic valve or Turner's syndrome.

258

CONGENITAL HEART DISEASE QUIZ

1. Bicuspid aortic valve occurs in approximately_____ of the population.
   a. 15-20%
   b. 20-30%
   c. 5-10%
   d. 1-2%

2. Coarctation of the aorta is usually located:
   a. proximal to the origin of the left subclavian artery
   b. proximal to the origin of the innominate artery
   c. in the mid descending aorta
   d. distal to the origin of the left subclavian artery

3. There are three basic types of subvalvular stenosis. A muscular deformity of the IVS in the subaortic region is classified as:
   a. Type I
   b. Type II
   c. Type III
   d. This is not a type of subvalvular stenosis

4. Supravalvular aortic stenosis is associated with:
   a. Eagle-Barrett syndrome
   b. William's syndrome
   c. Marfan's syndrome
   d. Down's syndrome

5. The process that allows the fetal heart to divide the expanding portions of the heart into four distinct chambers of the adult heart is referred to as:
   a. Cardiac looping
   b. Partitioning
   c. Cardiac septation
   d. Cardiac diverticulation

6. Pulmonic stenosis is often associated with:
   a. Ebstein's anomaly
   b. Marfan's syndrome
   c. Tetralogy of Fallot
   d. William's syndrome

7. The second most common form of congenital defect found in adults is:
   a. ventricular septal defects
   b. atrial septal defects
   c. Ebstein's anomaly
   d. Tetralogy of Fallot

8. Of all atrial septal defects, 70% are:
   a. ostium primum
   b. atrial secundum
   c. sinus venosus
   d. defects in the region of the coronary sinus

9. What type of atrial septal defect may be associated with abnormal drainage of the right pulmonary vein?
   a. ostium primum
   b. sinus venosus
   c. atrial secundum
   d. ostium sinus

10. Atrial septal defects that are of clinical significance are usually _____ or greater.
    a. 2 mm
    b. 1 mm
    c. 1 cm
    d. 3 cm

11. To calculate the pulmonary to systemic shunt ratio, which of the following is used?
    a. dp/dt
    b. CSA
    c. Qp/Qs
    d. SV/CO

12. The most common type of ventricular septal defect is:
    a. membranous
    b. muscular
    c. inlet
    d. outlet

13. Ventricular septal defects may be difficult to detect if they are less than:
    a. 10 mm
    b. 1 cm
    c. 5 mm
    d. 3 mm

14. Which of the following is NOT part of Eisenmenger's complex?
    a. ventricular septal defect
    b. pulmonary hypertension
    c. right ventricular hypertrophy
    d. mitral stenosis

15. A shunt from a patent ductus arteriosus will be noted from the:
    a. aorta to main pulmonary artery
    b. aorta to the right pulmonary artery
    c. aorta to IVC
    d. aorta to the SVC

16. Endocardial cushion defects have a high incidence with:
    a. Down's syndrome
    b. Marfan's syndrome
    c. acromegaly
    d. Fitz-Hugh-Curtis syndrome

17. Which of the following is NOT a part of a complete endocardial cushion defect?
    a. primum atrial septal defect
    b. ventricular septal defect
    c. cleft mitral valve
    d. cleft aortic valve
    e. cleft tricuspid valve

18. The leaflet of the tricuspid valve usually least affected by Ebstein's anomaly is the:
    a. septal
    b. posterior
    c. all affected the same
    d. anterior

19. A membranous ventricular septal defect, a large overriding aorta, and a right ventricular outflow tract obstruction are findings in what disease?
    a. Ebstein's anomaly
    b. Tetralogy of Fallot
    c. endocardial cushion defect
    d. Marfan's syndrome

20. An abnormal connection of the aorta and pulmonary artery to their respective ventricles describes:
    a. Truncus arteriosus
    b. Transposition of the great arteries
    c. Patent ductus arteriosus
    d. Patent foramen ovale

21. Diagnose the following image:
    a. right to left shunt
    b. left to right shunt
    c. mitral valve prolapse
    d. pericardial effusion

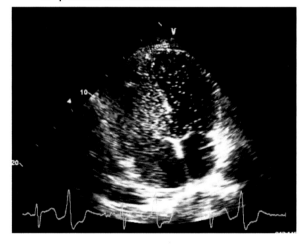

22. Diagnose the following image from the PSAX Aortic view:
    a. ASD
    b. VSD
    c. PDA
    d. MVP

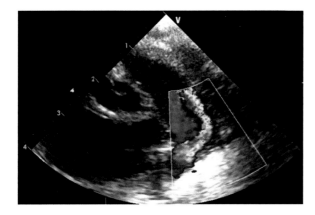

23. Bicuspid valves are best diagnosed during:
    a. Systole
    b. Diastole

24. A downward displacement of the TV causing the RV to become atrialized is known as:
    a. Ebstein's anomaly
    b. Eisenmenger's syndrome
    c. Dressler's syndrome
    d. Down's syndrome

25. Diagnose the following TEE image:
    a. ASD
    b. VSD
    c. PDA
    d. MVP

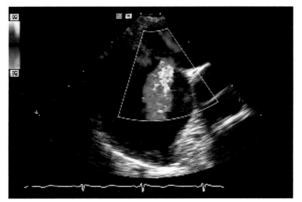

26. What type of a VSD is seen between 9 – 12 o'clock on the PSAX view of the Aorta?
    a. Outlet
    b. Perimembranous
    c. Trabecular
    d. Inlet

27. What is the RVSP with the given information:

    VSD peak velocity 4 m/sec
    BP 125/70

    a. 61 mmHg
    b. 75 mmHg
    c. 82 mmHg
    d. 90 mmHg

28. A Qp/Qs ratio greater than this number is considered significant and surgery is warranted:
    a. 1:1.5
    b. 1.5:1
    c. 1.5: 2.0
    d. 1.5: 1.5

29. Which type of TGA is typically cyanotic:
    a. L transposition
    b. D transposition
    c. C transposition
    d. M transposition

30. Coarctation of the Aorta is often associated with this abnormality:
    a. Bicuspid Aortic Valve
    b. ASD
    c. MVP
    d. Pericardial effusion

Section 11:

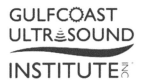

Diseases
of the Aorta

Section 11: DISEASES OF THE AORTA

Objectives:

Upon completion of this module you should be able to:

- Identify the common echocardiographic findings associated with Marfan's syndrome
- Recognize the various forms of aortic dilatation and their associated causes
- Apply the echocardiographic parameters used to evaluate the various diseases that can affect the aorta

Diseases of the Aorta

MARFAN'S SYNDROME

Marfan's syndrome is a hereditary disease of the fibrillin-1 gene resulting in abnormalities of connective tissue, bones, muscles, ligaments, and skeletal structures. Patients may exhibit arachnodactyly, pectus excavatum, aortic aneurysm, and mitral valve prolapse. The effects of Marfan's syndrome on the heart are manifested by aortic root enlargement or aneurysm, commonly at the level of the sinuses of Valsalva, but may be anywhere. Rupture of the aortic aneurysm can occur and surgical intervention is suggested when the aneurysm size exceeds 5.5cm.

Even though it is more common to have a dissection associated with an aneurysm, Marfan's patients may have an aortic dissection in the absence of an aneurysm. The anterior mitral leaflet is usually elongated and prolapses. Patients with a dilated aortic root may have varying degrees of aortic regurgitation. Mitral regurgitation may result as a consequence of the mitral valve prolapse.

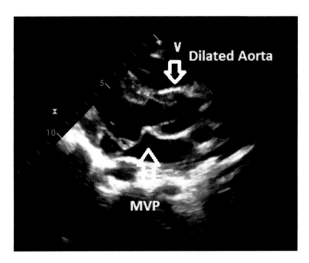

Marfan's Syndrome (Dilated Sinuses of Valsalva and Elongated Mitral Valve Leaflet)

AORTIC DILATATION

Aortic dilatation or enlargement is the most common aortic abnormality. The normal adult aorta at the root level should not exceed approximately 3.7 cm. Causes of aortic dilatation are: atherosclerosis, hypertension, cystic medial necrosis, post-stenotic dilatation, collagen-vascular diseases, and inflammation.

ANEURYSMS

Abnormal dilatation of the aorta is an aneurysm. Aneurysms can occur anywhere on the aorta. The most common causes are cystic medial necrosis, hypertension, atherosclerosis, Marfan's syndrome, collagen vascular disorders, and inflammatory diseases. Lesser causes of aortic aneurysms are tertiary syphilis, which is now uncommon in the United States, aortic arteritis, and blunt trauma. Depending on the location, aortic regurgitation of varying amounts may be present.

2-D imaging in the parasternal long and short axis views helps to visualize the ascending aorta and a portion of the descending aorta. Portions of the ascending aorta, arch, and descending can be seen from a suprasternal view, unfortunately, this view cannot be obtained on all patients.

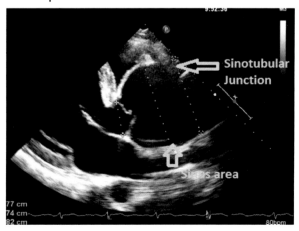

Aneurysm of Ascending Aorta

267

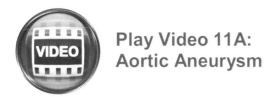 Play Video 11A:
Aortic Aneurysm

AORTIC DISSECTION

Aortic dissection is a result of the intima of the vessel wall pulling away from the media or middle layer of the arterial wall. An intimal flap, or false channel is formed between the tear and the vessel. Several complications can occur as a result of this: the false lumen can expand and compress the true lumen which supplies the arterial branches arising from the aorta, the intimal tear or flap can extend down the lumens of major arterial branches, thromboses can occur as a result of stasis of blood in the false lumen, and the vessel can rupture.

Causes of aortic dissection are associated with preexisting aneurysms, trauma, bicuspid or unicuspid valve disease, and chronic hypertension. Chronic hypertension is the most prevalent risk factor in patients with dissections. Patients with a unicuspid or bicuspid valve have an approximately five times higher incidence of dissection than normal patients. Aortic regurgitation and left ventricular dilatation may be associated findings.

Aortic dissections are classified according to the location and extent of the dissection in the aorta. The two most common classifications are the DeBakey and Stanford classifications.

The DeBakey classification breaks the dissections down to Types I, II, or III, III a and b.

DeBakey Classification of Aortic Dissection

Type I Intimal starts at the proximal ascending aorta and the dissection extends from the ascending aorta, arch, and portions of the descending and abdominal aorta.

Type II The dissection is only in the ascending aorta.

Type III The dissection may be limited to the descending thoracic aorta.
or
Type IIIa The dissection may involve the abdominal aorta and iliac vessels.

Type IIIb The dissection may involve the ascending aorta and arch.

Stanford Classification of Aortic Dissection

Type A All cases that involve the ascending aorta.

Type B All cases that involve the descending aorta.

Imaging of an aortic dissection may be technically limited on the transthoracic echocardiogram. Views of the aortic root and ascending aorta may be obtained from a variety of planes including the parasternal long and short axis, apical long and five chamber, subcostal and suprasternal views. Transesophageal echocardiography has proven to be an excellent means of assessing the aorta for the detection of a dissection and is considered by some to be just as accurate, if not more than CAT scan and aortography.

268

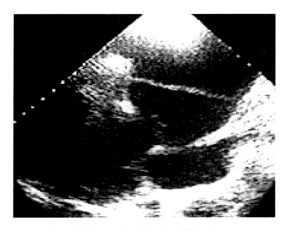

Aortic Dissection Proximal Aorta

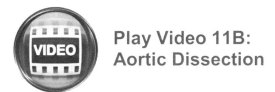

Play Video 11B:
Aortic Dissection

SINUS OF VALSALVA ANEURYSMS

Sinus of Valsalva aneurysms may be congenital or acquired. Causes include: infection, previous surgical procedures, and Marfan's syndrome. When the sinus of Valsalva has an aneurysm it protrudes into the adjacent chamber. A right coronary sinus aneurysm protrudes into the right ventricle, a left coronary sinus aneurysm protrudes into the left atrium, and the non-coronary sinus aneurysm protrudes into the right atrium. Rupture can occur and is usually the right coronary sinus.

It is unusual for a rupture to extend into the pericardium and is almost always fatal if it does. Symptoms may include: severe retrosternal pain, abdominal pain, and congestive heart failure. If a rupture has occurred, a diastolic murmur may be heard.

The basic 2-D views to visualize the sinuses of Valsalva are the parasternal long and short axis. Enlargement of the aortic root will be noted on both the 2-D and M-mode tracings. If aortic regurgitation

is present, the left ventricle may be enlarged. If a rupture into the right ventricle occurs, tricuspid systolic flutter may be noted. Other cardiac conditions that may be confused for an aneurysm of the sinus of Valsalva are: diverticulum of the anterior mitral valve leaflet, prolapse of the aortic cusp(s), prolapse of the anterior mitral valve leaflet, aneurysm of the membranous septum, aortic ring abscess, and other variations of the adjacent structures.

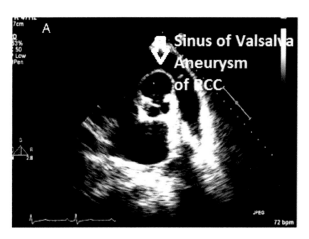

Sinus of Valsalva Aneurysm

COARCTATION OF THE AORTA

A narrowing of the descending aorta just distal to the left subclavian artery is referred to as coarctation of the aorta. Coarctation of the aorta may be responsible for hypertension and is associated with: bicuspid aortic valve, Turner syndrome, patent ductus arteriosus, aneurysm of the circle of Willis, and ventricular septal defects. The suprasternal view may be able to visualize the narrowing of the descending aorta, but if that is not possible, the defect can be detected by increased Doppler flow velocities at the site of the narrowing.

Another imaging modality that is helpful in the determination of coarctation of the aorta is MRI.

269

DISEASES OF THE AORTA QUIZ

1. A narrowing of the descending aorta just distal to the left subclavian artery is called:
    a. Marfans syndrome
    b. Sinus of Valsalva aneurysm
    c. coarctation
    d. type A dissection

2. The most common cause of aortic dissection is:
    a. Marfan's syndrome
    b. chronic hypertension
    c. unicuspid aortic valve
    d. trauma

3. The most common location to have a ruptured sinus of Valsalva is the:
    a. right ventricle
    b. left ventricle
    c. left atrium
    d. right atrium

4. The best view(s) for evaluating a sinus of valsalva aneurysm is/are:
    a. parasternal long axis
    b. parasternal short axis
    c. apical four chamber
    d. subcostal
    e. a & b
    f. b & d

5. Aortic dissection is best evaluated by:
    a. transthoracic echocardiography
    b. transesophageal echocardiography
    c. stress echocardiography
    d. pharmacologic stress echocardiography

6. Diagnose the following TEE image:
    a. Dissection of the aorta
    b. Mitral valve prolapse
    c. Mitral stenosis
    d. Myxoma

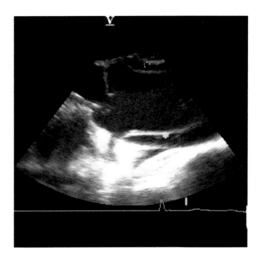

7. The normal adult aorta at the root level should not exceed ____cm.
    a. 1.5 cm
    b. 2.0 cm
    c. 2.5 cm
    d. 3.7 cm

8. What is the most likely cause for the following image:
    a. Systemic hypertension
    b. Dressler's syndrome
    c. Down's syndrome
    d. Marfan's syndrome

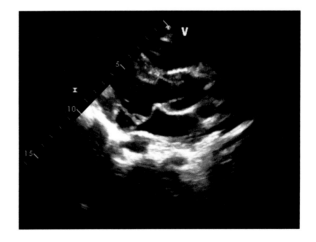

271

9. What type of Aortic dissection involves the descending aorta only:
    a. Debakey Type I
    b. Stanford Type A
    c. Debakey Type II
    d. Stanford Type B

10. The intimal flap in a dissection of the aorta at the ascending level may mimic this normal structure:
    a. Aortic valve
    b. Mitral valve
    c. Chordae tendineae
    d. Papillary muscle

Section 12:

Doppler

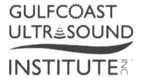

Section 12: DOPPLER

Objectives

Upon completion of this module you should be able to:

- State the general concept of the Doppler equation
- Cite the purpose of using the modified Bernoulli equation for echocardiography
- Apply the quantitative methods such as the pressure half-time formula to the cardiac Doppler examination
- Relate the pathologic findings associated with the various cardiac diseases to the color imaging and Doppler examination

DOPPLER

GENERAL INFORMATION

This section is an overview of Doppler and its applications in the heart since most of these aspects of Doppler have been discussed several times throughout this series and an in-depth discussion is provided in the *UltraPASS Sonography Physics and Instrumentation* companion workbook.

The Doppler effect can be described as a change in the observed frequency of sound, light, or other waves that is caused by motion of the source or of the observer.

The Doppler equation is:

$$V = \frac{c\,(+/-\,\Delta f)}{2fo\,(\cos\Theta)}$$

In this equation:

> **V** = flow velocity in meters per second.
> **C** = the speed of sound in tissue. The speed of sound in tissue is approximately 1540 meters per second.
> **+/- delta f** = Doppler frequency shift in hertz.
> **fo** = transmitted frequency
> **cosine Θ** = cosine function of the angle between the ultrasound beam and the blood flow velocity.

The **Doppler shift** is the difference between the transmitted frequency and detected frequency. A critical factor in accurate velocity calculation in the Doppler equation is the cosine of the angle. Interrogation should be performed as close to zero degrees (parallel) to flow to obtain the highest frequency shift.

Using these equations and physics principles, cardiac hemodynamics can be assessed accurately. Doppler can help to determine the timing, direction and quality of flow.

SPECTRAL ANALYSIS

The Doppler signal can be evaluated audibly (since Doppler shift falls within the audible range of 20-20,000 Hz) and/or displayed on a real time spectral analyzer. The Fast Fourier Transform (FFT) technique breaks down the mixture and range of signals, bands them together, and displays them as a function of time.

Spectral analysis allows us to visualize the range of Doppler frequencies present in a signal when Doppler shifts are detected simultaneously from reflectors moving at different speeds. The spectral display allows for evaluating blood flow direction, blood flow characteristics, quality of flow, and quantification of blood flow.

Flow direction in the heart is displayed based on the flow relative to the ultrasound beam. Blood flow that is moving towards the incoming ultrasound beam is referred to as antegrade flow and is depicted above the zero baseline on the Doppler spectral tracing. Flow that moves away from the incoming Doppler beam is referred to as retrograde flow and is displayed below the zero base.

When color flow imaging is being performed, the acronym BART applies to the depiction of flow direction relative to the ultrasound beam. BART means blue away, red towards, or flow away from the transducer is depicted in shades of blue and flow towards the transducer is depicted in shades of red.

The spectral tracing and color map are never inverted during cardiac Doppler unlike vascular Doppler. The optimum Doppler angle is 0 degrees to flow. This means that the ultrasound signal sent from the transducer needs to intersect blood flow at 0 degrees, or is parallel to flow. Doppler angles of greater than 20% lead to large errors in flow quantification

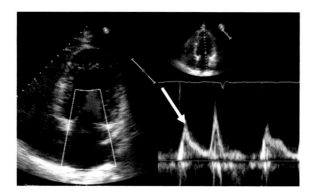

Spectral Tracing of Antegrade Flow

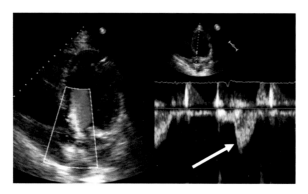

Spectral Tracing of Retrograde Flow

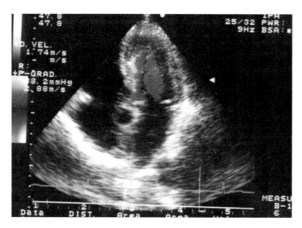

BART... Blue Away, Red Towards

DOPPLER INSTRUMENTS

Continuous Wave

Continuous wave Doppler utilizes two transducers. One crystal constantly transmits a signal while the second crystal continuously receives the reflected signal. This technique allows the examiner to evaluate high frequency flows (possibly stenotic lesions) at deep depths without experiencing any display artifacts (aliasing). Since the two transducers are constantly transmitting and receiving signals, the sound beams will overlap.

The region where the two beams overlap is called the **zone of sensitivity** and is the region where flow is detected. Blood flow will be detected along the entire beam path, resulting in a mixture of Doppler signals. If two vessels are located adjacent to one another, blood flow from both vessels will be detected. In addition, no range or depth resolution is provided.

Continuous wave Doppler is very useful in cardiac applications where the area of interest is usually at deep depths and high velocities are encountered in stenotic valves and other pathology. The duty factor (percentage of time the sound is on) in CW Doppler instruments is 1 or 100%.

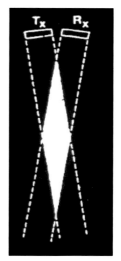

CW Doppler Transducer

278

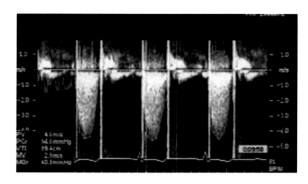

CW Waveform through Aortic Valve

The usual signal processing method used in CW Doppler is known as the **quadrature detection.** This employs two demodulators, located after the receiver (amplifier). The received signal is amplified and sent to these two demodulators, where two Doppler signals (output) are produced. These signals are mixed with two reference signals from the transmitter, respectively.

After filtering, the result is two almost identical Doppler signals, but they may differ in their phase. This difference is exactly one fourth (1/4) the period of the reference frequency. The difference in phase on the two output Doppler signals depends on whether the received echo signal frequency is greater or less than the transmitted signal frequency and depends on whether the scatters are moving toward or away from the transducer. This can be used to determine flow direction in directional CW Doppler instruments.

Pulsed Wave Doppler

Pulsed Doppler techniques utilize one crystal (or group of piezoelectric elements in the case of electronic arrays), which acts as the transmitter and receiver. The Doppler information measured in pulsed Doppler is detected by placing a sample gate or sample volume within a specific area in the heart or blood vessel. This technique gives the sonographer the ability to know what depth and anatomical area the blood flow is being detected from.

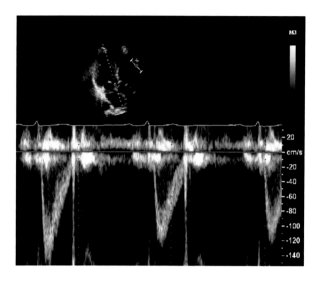

Pulsed Doppler

Unlike CW techniques, pulsed Doppler transmits a signal and then waits to receive the reflected signal before sending a second signal. This is called the **pulse repetition frequency or PRF** and denotes the number of pulses per second the system is sending to the area of interest. It is also called sampling or **pulsing rate.**

The transmit pulse length is determined by the sample volume length.

Long SV = long pulse length
Small SV = short transmit pulse

There are imaging and non-imaging pulsed Doppler instruments. A transcranial transducer is an example of a non-imaging pulsed Doppler Instrument. Duplex systems combine a real-time image with Doppler analysis.

279

Aliasing

The maximum Doppler shift a system can detect at a certain point in the display is called the **Nyquist limit** and is equal to one-half the PRF. In other words, the Nyquist sampling rate is when $PRF_{max} = 2f_D$. This limit defines the minimum sampling rate (PRF) for a signal whose frequency is f_D. If the sampling rate is *below* the Nyquist limit ($2f_D$), aliasing will occur. If it is *above* the Nyquist rate, the signal can be determined and displayed unambiguously. For example, if the PRF is 10 KHz, the maximum frequency shift the system can display in one direction is 5 KHz. If the received frequency shift exceeds 5 KHz, aliasing will occur.

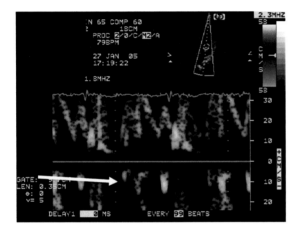

Aliasing

In any situation where sampling of a vessel occurs, the greater the sampling frequency (increased PRF) in comparison with the actual frequency present, the better the rendition of that signal after it has been sampled. Again, if detected frequencies (or velocities) increase in a way to overpass for two times the sampling frequency, an aliased signal occurs.

PW Doppler is limited in the display of high velocities at deep depths. Aliasing is presented in the display in different forms in spectral Doppler: first, the display "wraps- around" producing an apparent reversal of flow.

Second, in audible Doppler, there is a perception of loss of high frequencies as the frequency exceeds the maximum. It is important to realize that aliasing alone is <u>not</u> always diagnostic of severe disease, but simply reveals a display artifact. If velocity scale, angle, frequency, etc. for Doppler detection is set according to the vessel/heart physiology (velocities) and other diagnostic criteria for stenosis/pathology are present (B-Mode, etc.), then aliased signals need to be taken into consideration as indirect indicators of high-grade stenosis.

The sonographer can attempt to resolve aliasing by adjusting some controls on the system. These include:

- adjust the baseline shift
- increase the PRF (velocity range or scale)
- decrease the transmit frequency
- increase the incident angle

Baseline Shift: Changes the amount of display allotted to forward or reverse flow. Shifting the zero baseline **does not** affect the PRF.

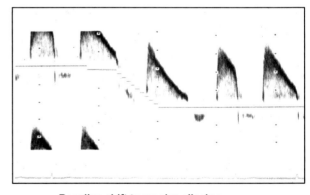

Baseline shift to resolve aliasing

Pulse Repetition Frequency (PRF) is the number of pulse echo cycles per second. Higher velocity flow detection requires higher PRF settings. Low velocity flow requires low PRF settings. PRF is also called velocity range or scale.

> **Rule of Thumb:**
> - **Use high PRF settings for high velocity flow**
> - **Use low PRF settings for low velocity flow**

To overcome maximum velocity limitations, some instruments provide a high PRF mode (HPRF). When high velocities need to be detected at large depths, the system can display the detected signals without ambiguity.

Caution must be used with HPRF Doppler as multiple sample volumes are active and can detect signals from nearby vessels or cardiac chambers.

Advantages/Disadvantages of CW & PW

The following table summarizes the advantages and disadvantages for both Pulsed Wave and Continuous Wave Doppler methods. Notice how the disadvantages of one technique become the advantages of the other

.

	CW	PW
Disadvantages	No duplex	Aliasing
	Range ambiguity	Cannot quantify High/deep velocities
	Inherent spectral broadening	
Advantages	No aliasing	Range resolution
	Quantify high/deep velocities	True Duplex
		Better characterize Blood flow I.e.turbulence

DOPPLER QUANTIFICATION

There are several parameters of flow that can be evaluated with Doppler echocardiography. The highest flow velocity through the valves can be determined by directing the Doppler signal at or slightly distal to the valve.

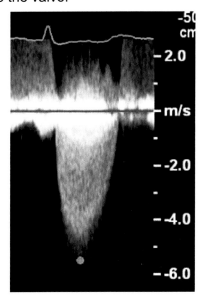

Doppler of Valve Velocity

Modified Bernoulli equation

If the valve is stenotic, a peak pressure gradient can be determined using the modified Bernoulli equation of:

$PPG = 4V^2$

V = the peak velocity of the blood flow. The pressure gradient is the pressure drop across an obstruction to flow.
The mean pressure gradient or average can also be obtained. The spectral Doppler is traced and the multiple velocities in the spectral envelope are converted into gradients and averaged. This is usually referred to as obtaining a VTI or TVI, velocity time integral, or time velocity integral.

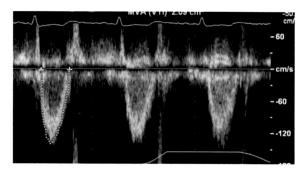

Doppler VTI/TVI

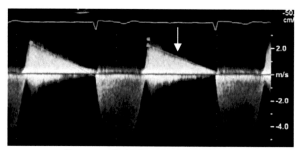

Pressure Half-time for Mitral Stenosis

Stroke Volume can be calculated using Doppler at any intracardiac site where the cross-sectional area and VTI can be recorded.

SV = CSA X VTI

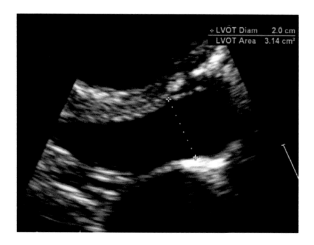

LVOT Diameter Measurement

Pressure Half-Time Formula

Valve area calculations of the mitral and tricuspid valve can be made using the pressure half-time formula.

MVA = 220/PHT

Pressure half-time is the time interval between the maximum early diastolic transmitted pressure gradient and the time point where the pressure gradient is half the maximum value.

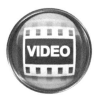

Play Video 12A: Mitral Flow

Pressure half-time can also be used to determine the severity of aortic regurgitation. When pressure half-time is used to calculated valve area, the higher the pressure half-time, the more severe the valvular stenosis. The opposite is true for aortic regurgitation. Lower pressure half- times indicate a higher degree of regurgitation. A pressure half-time of 200 msec would suggest severe aortic regurgitation.

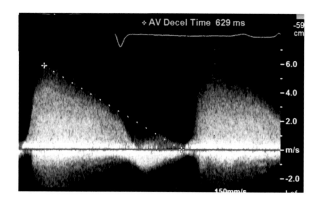

Pressure Half-time of Aortic Regurgitation

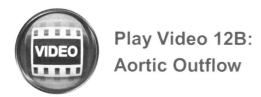

Play Video 12B:
Aortic Outflow

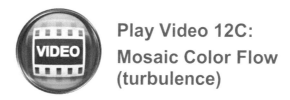

Play Video 12C:
Mosaic Color Flow
(turbulence)

The continuity equation can evaluate valve area. This equation is commonly applied to the aortic valve.

$$AVA = D^2 \times 0.785 \times \frac{VTI\ LVOT}{VTI\ AoV} =$$

$$\frac{SV}{VTI\ AoV}$$

COLOR FLOW MAPPING

Color flow imaging is pulsed Doppler technology that uses multiple sample gates along multiple scan lines to obtain frequency information. Autocorrelation is the digital technique used to analyze color flow Doppler. This information is color coded in shades of red and blue. Flow towards the transducer is displayed in red shades and flow away from the transducer is displayed in blue shades.

This information is superimposed over the 2-D image to represent blood flow. The color encoding is also depicted on the color bar along with the velocity scale. Color flow imaging allows for detection of flow and hemodynamic consequences of disease.

Turbulent flow often has a mosaic effect where colors of red, yellow, blue and cyan are seen. These colors and their changes help to provide information regarding valvular regurgitation and stenosis, congenital defects, and other abnormal flow states.

With color flow imaging there may be a tendency to overestimate disease severity due to the colorization of flow, especially with the beginner sonographer.

Color flow imaging is limited to good visualization of the heart and good Doppler angle. Arrhythmias, bradycardia, and tachycardia can also affect the color exam.

Frame rate may be one of the most important technical factors used to optimize color flow imaging. This is controlled by the size of the color box or sector. A wider sector or box decreases the frame rate, therefore decreasing resolution. A longer sector or box decreases the pulse repetition frequency also effecting resolution. The optimum sector or color box size is one that is large enough to cover the area of interest, but does not limit resolution.

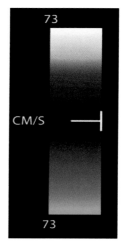

Velocity Scale

DOPPLER QUIZ

1. In the Doppler equation the C represents:
   a. velocity of flow
   b. Doppler frequency shift
   c. transmitted frequency
   d. speed of sound in tissue

2. The difference between the transmitted frequency and the detected frequency is:
   a. Nyquist limit
   b. PRF
   c. Doppler shift
   d. Reynolds number

3. The best Doppler angle to blood flow is:
   a. 10 degrees
   b. 20 degrees
   c. 0 degrees
   d. 90 degrees

4. A peak pressure gradient of flow through a valve is obtained by using the equation:
   a. $4V^2$
   b. squared 4
   c. PHT/220
   d. $V4^2$

5. A pressure half-time measurement is used to evaluate:
   a. aortic stenosis
   b. mitral stenosis
   c. mitral regurgitation
   d. aortic regurgitation
   e. a & c
   f. b & d

6. To calculate aortic valve area, which one of the following equations can be used?
   a. Bernoulli equation
   b. continuity equation
   c. pressure half-time
   d. modified Simpson's

7. One of the most important technical factors used to optimize color flow images besides proper Doppler angle is:
   a. gain
   b. frame rate
   c. Nyquist limit
   d. Variance

8. Color flow imaging uses ____Doppler.
   a. pulsed
   b. continuous wave

9. The velocity time integral measurement calculates:
   a. peak pressure gradient
   b. mean pressure gradient
   c. aortic valve area
   d. mitral valve area

10. The formula CSA x VTI is used to calculate:
    a. mean pressure gradient
    b. peak pressure gradient
    c. stroke volume
    d. pressure half-time

11. The following image represents:
    a. stenosis
    b. aliasing
    c. color flow
    d. high flow

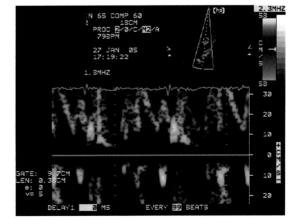

12. The following image represents:
    a. blue away red toward
    b. blue stenosis red regurgitation
    c. blue towards red away
    d. blue regurgitation red stenosis

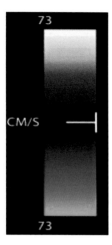

13. Reflected frequency is higher than transmitted frequency:
    a. positive Doppler shift
    b. negative Doppler shift
    c. no Doppler shift
    d. Doppler change

14. Methods to avoid aliasing include:
    a. shifting baseline
    b. decrease depth
    c. switch to CW
    d. all of the above

Section 13:

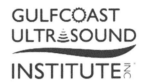

Stress Echocardiography

Section 13: STRESS ECHOCARDIOGRAPHY

Objectives

Upon completion of this module you should be able to:

- Cite the applications of stress echo

- Perform routine procedures associated with stress echo

- Apply the basic concepts of stress echo

- Relate knowledge of ischemic heart disease to stress echo

STRESS ECHOCARDIOGRAPHY

The primary goal in stress echocardiography is to help identify patients with coronary insufficiency. Stress echocardiography, like other forms of stress testing, is a screening tool. The "gold standard" for identifying coronary anatomy and the presence of coronary artery disease is angiography.

Indications for Stress Testing

- Identification of severe coronary artery disease
- Diagnosis of myocardial disease
- Preoperative evaluation
- Determine risk level post-acute myocardial infarction

There are several factors that determine the type of stress testing that best suits the patient.

FACTORS DETERMINING TYPE OF STRESS TESTING

- Patient size (weight)
- Patient's ability to exercise
- Clinical issues
- Resting ECG (EKG)
- Expertise associated with testing

Stress echocardiography can be accomplished through a variety of methods. Exercise can be performed on a treadmill or bicycle, or the heart can be stressed with the use of pharmacologic agents, or transesophageal atrial pacing.

All stress echocardiograms begin with a set of resting images of the heart. These digitized images can easily be stored, displayed, and retrieved. Capturing of the images is triggered by the QRS complex on the EKG.

Four views are typically obtained during systole with stress echocardiography. They are the parasternal long and short axis, and the apical four and two chamber views. The short axis view is most commonly obtained at the level of the papillary muscles. The initial resting images are stored to be compared.

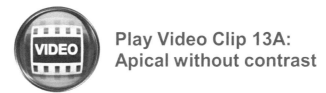

Play Video Clip 13A: Apical without contrast

When stress echocardiography is performed using a treadmill to exercise the patient, the post exercise images should be obtained within the first 60 - 90 seconds after exercise has stopped. Most labs try to obtain images within the first 60 seconds.

The ability to obtain these images as quickly as possible increases the accuracy of the exam since wall motion abnormalities may last for only a few minutes after exercise. After the post exercise images are obtained, they are placed on a quad-screen display adjacent to the same view obtained at rest.

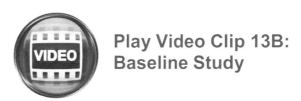

Play Video Clip 13B: Baseline Study

If an upright or supine bicycle is used to perform the stress test, the images are obtained during peak exercise. This technique may be more technically limiting due to patient movement and poor cardiac windows.

Pharmacologic agents can be used to induce stress when a patient is unable to do so. Medications that are used to induce stress are: dobutamine, dipyridamole, and adenosine. Atropine can be used if the target heart rate is not achieved at the maximum dose of dobutamine. Atropine is typically given at a dose of 0.5 mg – 1.0 mg every minute until HR is achieved.

Imaging may be performed during pre, low dose, mid dose and peak administration of the drug. Some labs may do pre, low dose, high dose and post. Patients that are on beta blockers may not be able to reach an adequate heart rate, so atropine may be given. The wall motion is compared from level to level including the baseline images. Ischemia may not be manifested in the same way during Dobutamine stress as it is during exercise stress.

During regular exercise stress testing severe coronary artery disease may cause the left ventricle to dilate, the ejection fraction decreases, ST-depression on the EKG is common, and hypotension may result. These findings may not be found, or are not specific when Dobutamine is used to induce stress.

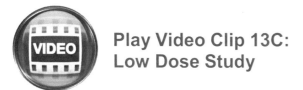

Play Video Clip 13C: Low Dose Study

The obvious indication of an abnormal stress echocardiogram is the detection of a wall motion abnormality that was not present on the resting exam. If a wall motion abnormality was present, the next step is to determine if it got worse. A hypokinetic wall that becomes akinetic, or an akinetic wall that becomes dyskinetic is an indication of ischemia. If the wall motion abnormality does not change, then the wall may be infarcted. When akinetic wall motion abnormalities improve after exercise, then the myocardium may be viable.

TECHNICAL CONSIDERATIONS

- Optimize image before stress.
- If patient develops chest pain, or the ECG indicates significant changes during recovery, additional dynamic images should be acquired and stored.
- Try to obtain the easiest views first, if all views are easy, perform the apical images first.
- Do not adjust the image depth during the exam, keep it the same for all of the images.

Stress echocardiography may be used to assess the hemodynamics in valvular heart disease. When clinical symptoms do not correlate with measurements performed at rest, stress echocardiography may be helpful.

Stress echocardiography may be contraindicated on patients with severe aortic stenosis and poor left ventricular systolic function. All stress testing should be carefully monitored, but especially when being performed on patients with valvular heart disease.

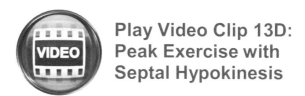

Play Video Clip 13D: Peak Exercise with Septal Hypokinesis

Contrast agents have been a great success in the field of echocardiography and stress testing. Diagnostic images could not be obtained in up to 30% of the patients that were sent for stress echocardiography. New contrast agents have improved imaging and the detection of the endocardial border up to 95%. Better image quality through the use of contrast agents and harmonic imaging has led to increased diagnostic accuracy, and hopefully, a more cost-effective method to evaluate the heart.

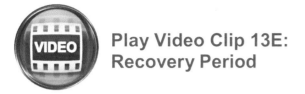 **Play Video Clip 13E: Recovery Period**

STRESS ECHO QUIZ

1. The optimum time to capture images after a treadmill exercise stress test is:
   a. 1 minute
   b. 5 minutes
   c. 3 minutes
   d. 4 minutes

2. The "gold standard" for the determination of ischemic heart disease is:
   a. stress ECG
   b. stress echocardiogram
   c. PET scan
   d. angiography

3. Which steps are recommended to ensure the BEST quality stress echocardiogram?
   a. Optimize images before stressing the patient
   b. Keep same depth and contrast for pre and post images
   c. Perform tissue Doppler on pre and post images
   d. Use of contrast improves visualization of segments in up to 95% of patients
   e. all of the above

4. During a pharmacologic stress test, images should be acquired during: the following stages:
   a. low and high dose only
   b. low dose and peak dose only
   c. pre, low dose, mid dose, and peak
   d. pre peak dose only

5. When an akinetic area of the heart becomes hypokinetic after exercise, the cardiac tissue may be:
   a. infarcted
   b. viable
   c. stunned
   d. hibernating

6. What drug can be given to patients on beta blockers when Dobutamine does not achieve an adequate heart rate?
   a. adenosine
   b. atropine
   c. Dipyridamole
   d. thallium

7. When should image acquisition begin during bicycle exercise stress test?
   a. immediately after exercise has stopped
   b. during peak exercise
   c. after peak exercise
   d. 90 seconds after exercise has stopped

8. Which of the following is NOT a positive finding on an exercise stress echocardiogram?
   a. normal to hypokinetic wall motion
   b. hypokinetic to akinetic wall motion
   c. akinetic to dyskinetic wall motion
   d. normal to hyperdynamic wall motion

9. Beta blockers may prohibit attaining peak heart rate in Pharmacologic Stress Echo:

   True or False

10. An indication for a stress echo would be:
    a. chest pain with exercise
    b. congestive heart failure
    c. aortic stenosis
    d. all of the above

ALL SECTION QUIZ ANSWERS

Section 1:
Anatomy and
Physiology
1. d
2. c
3. b
4. d
5. b
6. a
7. c
8. c
9. e
10. d
11. d
12. c
13. a
14. b
15. d
16. c
17. b
18. c
19. c
20. d
21. a
22. e
23. c
24. d
25. c
26. b
27. a
28. c
29. d
30. a
31. c
32. a
33. c
34. a
35. c
36.

O Mitral valve closure

Atrial systole O   O Ventricular repolarizatic

Aortic valve opening

37. b
38. d
39. b
40. c
41. b

42. b
43. a
44. d

Section 2:
Technique
1. c
2. b
3. b
4. c
5. a
6. c
7. b
8. c
9. b
10. b
11. d
12. a
13. a
14. b
15. c
16. d
17. d
18. b
19. a
20. c
21. b
22. d
23. b
24. c
25. d
26. b
27. c
28. c
29. a
30. c
31. b
32. c
33. a
34. c
35. a
36. b
37. b
38. b
39. a
40.   1) RCC
     2) LV
     3) LA
     4) Antero-septal wall

41. c
42. c

43. c
44. b
45. b
46. c
47. d
48. b
49. c
50. c
51. b

Section 3:
Valvular Heart
Disease
1. d
2. a
3. b
4. d
5. c
6. c
7. b
8. b
9. c
10. b
11. c
12. a
13. b
14. a
15. d
16. a
17. b
18. d
19. b
20. c
21. a
22. b
23. d
24. b
25. b
26. a
27. a
28. a
29. a
30 c.
31. b
32. c
33. b
34. a
35. a
36. c
37. b
38. c
39. b

40. c
41. a
42. d
43. c
44. a
45. c
46. c
47. d
48. b
49. c
50. d
51. c
52. b
53. c
54. d
55. b
56. c
57. b
58. b
59. c
60. d
61. b
62. b
63. c
64. b
65. d
66. c
67. d
68. c
69. c
70. b
71. b
72.
a) > 1.5 m/sec peak MV velocity
d) >8 cm^2 Regurgitant jet area
f) 40% RJA/LAA

73. b
74. b
75. b,d,f,g
    b)Radius
    d) MR Peak
      Velocity
    f) MR VTI
    g) Aliasing Velocity

76. c
77. c
78. a

**Section 4:
Pericardial
Disease**
1. d
2. c
3. b
4. a
5. b
6. b
7. b
8. b
9. b
10. b
11. d
12. c
13. c
14. c
15. d
16. d
17. d
18. c
19. a
20. a
21. a
22. b
23. c
24. c
25. c
26. b
27. c
28. b

**Section 5:
Systemic and
Pulmonary HTN**
1. c
2. d
3. d
4. c
5. f
6. e
7. a
8. c
9. d
10. c
11. d
12. c
13. b
14. d
15. c
16. c
17. a
18. b

**Section 6:
Cardiomyopathies**
1. c
2. d
3. d
4. b.
5. b
6. c
7. c
8. c

9. a
10. d
11. a
12. d
13. b
14. b
15. d
16. e
17. c
18. a
19. c
20. a
21. a
22. d
23. d
24. a
25. b
26. c
27. b
28. d
29. b
30. c
31. b
32. b
33. d
34. a
35. d
36. b
37. b
38. c
39. e
40. b
41. a
42. c
43. c
44. c
45. d
46. d

**Section 7: LV
Function**
1. c
2. a
3. c
4. b
5. a
6. b
7. e
8. e
9. c
10. d
11. c
12. c
13. c
14. c
15. d
16. a
17. b
18. d
19. d
20. a
21. c
22. b
23. b

24. d
25. b
26. d
27. d
28. c
29. d
30. c

**Section 8: Cardiac
Tumors**
1. c
2. c
3. b
4. a
5. d
6. c
7. f
8. f
9. a
10. e
11. b
12. b
13. d
14. b
15. d
16. d
17. c
18. b
19. a
20. Lipoma
    Fibroma
    Teratoma

**Section 9:
Miscellaneous**
1. c
2. b
3. c
4. a
5. a
6. c
7. d
8. c
9. a
10. d
11. e
12. d
13. d
14. a
15. a
16. c
17. c
18. c
19. b
20. a
21. b
22. d
23. c
24. b
25. a
26. d
27. a
28. c

Section 10: CHD
1. d
2. d
3. b
4. b
5. c
6. c
7. b
8. b
9. b
10. c
11. c
12. a
13. d
14. d
15. a
16. a
17. d
18. d
19. b
20. b
21. a
22. c
23. a
24. a
25. a
26. b
27. a
28. b
29. b
30. a

**Section 11:
Disease of the
Aorta**
1. c
2. b
3. a
4. e
5. b
6. a
7. d
8. d
9. d
10. a

**Section 12:
Doppler**
1. d
2. c
3. c
4. a
5. f
6. b
7. b
8. a
9. b
10. c
11. b
12. a
13. a
14. d

298

Section 13:
Stress Echo
1. a
2. d
3. d
4. c
5. b
6. b
7. b
8. d
9. True
10. a

REFERENCES

Aehlert, B. ECG Made Easy, 5th Edition, 2012, Mosby

Kremkau, F. Diagnostic Ultrasound: Principles and Instruments, 8th Edition, 2010, Saunders

Opie,L/ Gersh, B. Drugs for the Heart, 8th Edition, 2013, Saunders

Otto, C. Textbook of Clinical Echocardiography, 5th Edition, 2013, Saunders

Reynolds, T. The Echocardiographer's Pocket Reference, 4th Edition, 2013, Arizona Heart Institute

Tortora, G. Principles of Anatomy and Physiology, 14th Edition, 2013, Wiley

CME Certificate Instructions

To take the quiz for this program and receive CME credit:

1. Point your browser to https://www.gcus.com

2. Log into your account.

3. Select "My Activities" from the top menu, find this product **(PAU-OL6-CTP3)**, and click the "CME QUIZ/CREDIT" button to access your Pre-Paid Quiz, or purchase CME Quiz/Credit at this point.

4. Take the quiz.

5. After passing the quiz with a 70% or higher, fill out a short survey to continue.

6. A certificate will automatically be generated for you to print out.

Questions? Call (727)363-4500
Monday-Friday 8:30am-5:00pm EST